W9-CTU-947

INFORMED

AN INTRODUCTION TO MEDICAL SELF-CARE AND STAYING WELL

George J. Pfeiffer, M.S.E.
Allen Douma, M.D.

CONTENT REVIEWERS

William Hettler, M.D.

Michael Morse, M.D.

Michael Pfeiffer, D.D.S.

Steven Schmitz, M.D., M.P. H.

Barrie Gleason Carveth, R.N.

Judith Webster, R.N., M.S.

Scott Campbell, M.S.

Robin Foust

Jennifer Gleckman

Robert Larsen

Garry M. Lindsay, M. P. H., C.H.E.S.

Jan Murnane, M.Ed., M.B.A.

Elin Silveous

Published by WorkCare Press
The WorkCare Group, Inc.
Charlottesville, Virginia
First Edition

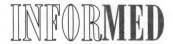

WorkCare Press

P.O. Box 2053
Charlottesville, Virginia 22902

ISBN Number: 0-9634986-0-6
Printed in the United States of America

PUBLISHER:	George J. Pfeiffer
EDITOR:	Sara Piccini
GRAPHICS AND DESIGN:	Steven and Sally Black
	Valerie L'Herrou
PRODUCTION MANAGER:	Paxson MacDonald
PROOFREADER:	Amy Lemley
INTERNAL ILLUSTRATIONS:	Sally Black
	Katherine Rose Crowther
Cover Illustration:	Ron Chan

Distributed in the United States by The WorkCare Group, Inc.
For sales inquiries and special prices for bulk quantities, write to the address above or call
The WorkCare Group, Inc., at (804) 977-7525.

Limits of Liability: *INFORMED: An Introduction to Medical Self-Care and Staying Well* **is intended to increase awareness of health and medical care issues. None of the information in this text is intended to be a substitute for appropriate physician diagnosis and medical care.**

CONTENTS

There is perhaps no more important issue in America today than health care. Everyone agrees that health care costs too much. People are afraid that one major accident or illness will wipe out their life savings.

Studies show that up to 25 percent of all health care costs are wasted through unnecessary medical tests and procedures, the inappropriate use of hospitalization and emergency room services, and doctor's visits for uncomplicated medical complaints such as colds and flu that could be treated through medical self-care.

In response to this epidemic of runaway costs and unnecessary procedures, there has been a greater movement toward *managed care systems*. Managed care systems use networks (e.g., HMOs) of physicians and hospitals to control health care costs through more appropriate use of medical services. Although managed care is a step in the right direction, the solution to our health care problems doesn't rest solely with physicians or insurance companies. *The solution begins with you through informed health care decision-making.*

How Well Are You Managing Your Health?

You may feel that dealing with the medical care system is beyond your control, or feel intimidated by medical terms, medical technology and talking to your doctor. *Today you can no longer afford to be just a passive patient in someone else's care. You need to be an "informed" decision-maker, capable of managing all aspects of your health and well-being.* This includes the day-to-day decisions you and your family make in trying to *prevent* illness and injury and decisions regarding the use of the medical care system.

Regardless of your health status, be it well or ill, it's important to be actively involved and informed in your health care decisions. This includes:

• Knowing and practicing life-style and self-care skills that help prevent and/or manage life-style related disorders.

• Being able to select a doctor based on your needs.

• Having the basic skills to know when medical care is necessary and when common problems can be treated at home.

• Being able to talk to your doctor comfortably, including questioning available treatment options and their benefits, risks and costs.

• Making joint decisions with your doctor on the need for hospitalization when outpatient services may be just as effective.

• Knowing your rights as a patient.

How INFORMED Can Help You

INFORMED is designed to give you a basic introduction to the principles of prevention, medical self-care and medical consumerism. Using this book will help you:

• Prevent and/or manage major problems such as heart disease, diabetes and cancer through positive lifestyle practices.

• Learn to treat common medical complaints through medical self-care.

• Reduce unnecessary medical tests, procedures and hospitalization.

• Reduce your out-of-pocket medical expenses.

• Have greater confidence and skills in dealing with medical care decisions.

• Have greater health and vitality.

We encourage you and your family to become familiar with your medical self-care options. When faced with a medical problem, make consulting this book your first step. However, this book is not intended to replace professional medical treatment when it's required or replace treatment already recommended by your health care provider. If you have any questions or concerns, consult your doctor first.

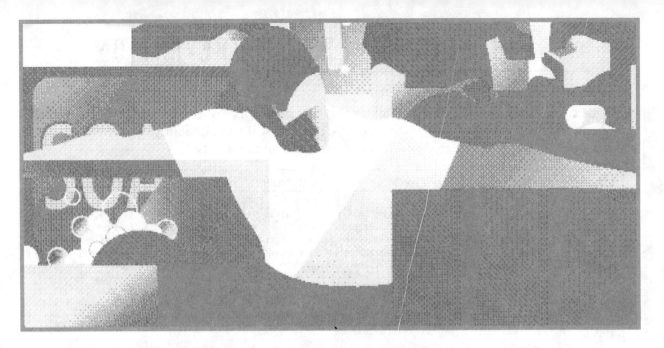

An Ounce Of Prevention

By Using This Section You Will:

• Learn what behaviors have the greatest influence in reducing your risk of illness and disease.

• Learn how to make regular exercise a part of your life.

• Learn how to eat right for good health.

• Learn 15 ways to reduce stress and tension in your life.

• Learn specific skills for losing weight and keeping it off.

• Learn how to have more energy in your life.

• Learn what medical screening tests are appropriate for you.

• Learn what immunizations are appropriate for you and family members.

P R E V E N T I O N

6

The cornerstone of health is practicing appropriate behaviors that not only increase your vitality and independence, but also help reduce the risk of disease and disability. The chart below lists behaviors that have the greatest influence on health and longevity.

BUILDING BLOCK	IDEAS THAT WORK	BENEFITS	RESOURCES
Staying Active	• Exercise 3 to 5 days per week, 20 to 60 minutes per session. • Uninterrupted activities involving large muscles, e.g.,walking, cycling and swimming are recommended. • Also, try resistance exercises that strengthen the shoulders, arms, back, abdomen and leg muscles. Recommended twice a week.	• Protects against heart disease, cancer, diabetes, osteoporosis, and depression. • Best for weight control. • Increases your energy level. • Maintains adequate levels of muscular strength and endurance needed to perform everyday activities.	• Local YMCA/YWCA • Recreation centers • Health clubs • Company fitness center • Home "gym" • American Heart Association, "Walking for a Healthy Heart"
Eating Right	• Keep total fat intake below 30 percent of total calories per day. • Limit saturated fat to less than 10 percent of total calories. • Consume 55 to 60 percent of total calories in carbohydrates. • Protein should be below 15 percent. Eat leaner cuts of red meat and substitute with fish (unfried) and poultry. • Eat more fruits, vegetables and grains. • Moderate your use of salt (sodium).	• Protects against heart disease, hypertension, cancer, diabetes and obesity. • Provides energy for mental and physical activities.	• American Cancer Society • American Dietetic Association • Refer to "Food Pyramid' on p. 11. • Refer to Five-A-Day Plan on p. 10. • American Heart Association
Watching Your Weight	• Keep your weight within 10 percent of ideal. • Avoid crash diets. • Increase your physical activity. • Reduce your total intake of fat. •Substitute high-fat foods with low-fat foods.	• Improves appearance. • Reduces risk of heart disease, hypertension and diabetes. • Reduces stress on joints. • Enhances self-esteem/self-image.	• American Dietetic Association • Refer to p. 13.
Drinking Alcohol In Moderation Or Not At All	• If you do drink, maximum of 1 to 2 drinks per day. • Don't drink and drive. • Don't operate equipment or machinery while under the influence of alcohol.	• Lowers risk of liver disease and certain cancers. • Reduces risk of on-the-job accidents and motor vehicle accidents.	• Your company employee assistance program (EAP) • Alcoholics Anonymous • Refer top. 103.

BUILDING BLOCK	IDEAS THAT WORK	BENEFITS	RESOURCES
Staying Drug-Free	• Use prescription and over-the-counter medications only as directed. • Don't use illicit drugs.	• Prevents dependence on drugs • Helps prevent the spread of AIDS.	• Narcotics Anonymous • Refer to p. 107.
Practicing Safe Sex	• Seek monogamous relationships. • Use condoms with the spermicide nonoxynol-9.	• Helps prevent sexually transmitted diseases such as HIV/AIDS, gonorrhea and chlamydia.	• Your personal physician • Local health department • Refer to p. 117.
Using Your Seat Belt	• Use your seat belt and shoulder harness 100 percent of the time. • Have all passengers buckle up before you start your vehicle. • If you have an infant, use child safety seats. Secure child in *back seat*.	• Reduces vehicular death and injury.	• National Safety Council • Local police
Following Scheduled Immunizations And Medical Tests	• Follow recommended schedules based on age, sex and health status.	• Identifies health risk • Prevents and/or manages disease. • Prevents infectious diseases.	• Your personal physician • Immunizations, p. 21. • Medical Tests, p. 19.
Staying Out Of The Sun	• Avoid sun during peak hours. • Apply sunscreen: SPF 15 or higher. • Cover up, wear a hat and other protective clothing.	• Prevents skin cancer. • Prevents premature aging.	• American Cancer Society

WALKING: THE BEST EXERCISE?

Whether you want to lose weight, manage stress or reduce your health risks, walking is perhaps the best way to add regular exercise to your life. Walking is inexpensive, needs little equipment, can be done almost anywhere and is good for young and old alike. Here are a few tips on starting your own walking program.

IDEAS THAT WORK:

- **Use the proper footwear.** Sneakers and running shoes may not give you adequate support and cushioning. There are several "walking shoes" on the market that are designed to help the heel-to-toe motion of walking and provide good support for the heel. When fitting your shoes, make sure that you have room in the front (toe box), allowing the toes to spread out as you push off from the ground.

- **Use proper form.** Walk erect, but keep your upper body relaxed. Foot contact with the ground should be heel to toe. You should feel a gentle rocking motion as you transfer your weight from your heel to the final push-off with your toes. You should hold your arms at a 90-degree angle, and swing them vigorously forward and back to help maintain momentum. Avoid crossing your arms in front of your chest, especially if you use hand weights.

- **Map your course.** To ensure personal safety and increase enjoyment, find a walking route that is out of the way of traffic, offers pleasant scenery, has an even surface, and is safe and well lit at night. Nearby shopping malls are excellent places to walk, especially in winter climates.

- **Start on the right foot.** If you are over 40 years old and have been inactive or, regardless of your age, have a medical condition such as high blood pressure, heart disease or joint problems, discuss your exercise plans with your doctor before starting. Begin your program slowly. Gradually increase the time (duration) of your walk before increasing the speed (intensity).

- **Buddy up!** You don't have to walk alone. Walk with a family member, friend or co-worker. Ideally, try to walk with someone at your fitness level.

- **Schedule your walk.** If it's been hard for you to exercise because you haven't had the time, schedule your walk and make it a habit. When was the last time you did something for yourself?

- **Add variety.** Though it's wise to have a regular walking route, try to vary your walking course once you've reached a level of comfort and regularity. Map out additional walking routes that vary in distance, terrain, and scenery, and are safe.

- **Start slowly, then build.** To begin feeling health benefits, walk a minimum of five days a week, for 30 minutes at a time. You may find that you can walk for only 10 minutes before needing a rest. Try joining three 10-minute walks with three-minute rest periods in between. Over time, increase your walking interval from 10 minutes to 13 minutes to 15 minutes and so on, or decrease the rest interval until you can walk the entire time. A rule of thumb is that if you can carry on a normal conversation without being out of breath, then you are exercising at an acceptable level of effort.

- **Move it, lose it.** If weight loss is your goal, research suggests that you need to walk for

WALKING: THE BEST EXERCISE?

at least 40 minutes five days per week to experience significant results. Studies have also shown that walking for 20 to 40 minutes seems to be the threshold for reducing anxiety and tension.

- **Refresh yourself.** On hot, humid days, be sure to drink at least 12 ounces of water before starting. It's also wise to carry a water bottle while exercising and drink before you become thirsty. On sunny days it's a good idea to use sunscreen and wear a brimmed hat and sunglasses.

- **Have fun!** Once you reach a level of activity that is comfortable, vary your walking routes, change the distance, play with the tempo, plan a picnic at the turnaround, walk through city parks or botanical gardens, have a company noon-hour walk program or participate in a community "walkathon" for charity.

- **Reward yourself or your walking group.** Establish an incentive program for your progress or set up an office walking or family fund. For every mile walked, contribute to the "walk fund." Once the fund has reached a certain amount, treat the group to movie tickets or lunch at a local restaurant, or donate the money to charity.

Walking Through The Day:

- *Ride and Walk: If you commute by mass transit, get off earlier than your usual stop and walk the additional distance.*

- *Park and Walk: Park your car farther from your place of work or at the back of the parking lot.*

- *Break Walk: Instead of running to the vending machine or smoking an extra cigarette, get out of the office and walk during your scheduled breaks.*

- *Lunch and Walk: If you "brown bag," walk to a nearby park that's five to seven minutes from the office. Sit and enjoy your lunch and walk back.*

- *Form a Walking Group: Form a noon-hour walking group. Have members alternate in choosing the route of the day.*

- *Walk After Dinner: Take a stroll for 20 to 30 minutes by yourself or with family member(s).*

RESOURCES:

Fitness Walking, by Robert Sweetgall. New York: Perigree Books, 1985.

Rockport Walking Program, by James M. Rippe. Englewood Cliffs, N.J.: Prentice-Hall, 1989.

F.Y.I. *The American College of Sports Medicine (ACSM) recommends that adults exercise three to five days per week in activities that encourage aerobic (with oxygen) conditioning for 20 to 60 minutes per session. Aerobic activities include brisk walking, jogging, cycling, aerobic dance and swimming. ACSM also recommends that strengthening exercises that condition major muscle groups (e.g. arms, shoulders, back and legs) be done twice a week. The important point to keep in mind are that regardless of what activity you choose to do— be regular, don't overdo it and enjoy yourself!*

P R E V E N T I O N

10

The National Institutes of Health recommends that diet be the first line of defense for prevention of heart disease and some cancers. The following nutritional guidelines are based on information from the American Heart Association, the American Cancer Society and the United States Dietary Guidelines.

FOOD FOR THOUGHT:

- **Build a pyramid.** The U.S government recently released a "Food Pyramid" that outlines the recommended daily servings of key food groups. This model suggests that we eat more breads, cereals, fruits and vegetables and less meat, dairy and fatty foods in order to reduce our risk of heart disease, cancer, diabetes and obesity. Refer to the Food Pyramid on p. 11.

- **Reduce fat.** Cut down on the amount of fat you eat, especially saturated fats found in marbled red meats, whole milk, many cheeses (e.g., cheddar and brie), and coconut and palm oils. The more fat you cut out of your diet, the more calories you save and the lower your risk of heart disease, obesity and cancer.

  – *Choose lean meats, poultry and fish.*

  - *Increase your consumption of fish and skinless poultry to two to three servings per week.*

  - *Trim away visible fat.*

  - *Try low-fat cooking methods such as broiling, baking and steaming.*

  - *When oils are needed, use those with monounsaturated fat such as canola and olive oils.*

  - *Substitute high-fat foods with lower-fat foods. Refer to p. 14.*

- **Cut the "Big C."** Control your intake of cholesterol-rich foods. Limit your consumption of animal fats, organ meats (such as liver), lobster, shrimp and eggs to reduce your risk of heart disease.

- **Add more high-fiber foods to your diet to protect against colon cancer.** Eat more whole grains, fruits, vegetables, wheat and whole-bran cereals, rice, popcorn and whole-wheat bread.

- **Reduce salt.** Limit salt-cured, smoked and nitrite-cured foods, and sodium laden processed foods and snacks.

- **Moderate your alcohol.** If you drink alcohol, limit your intake to fewer than two drinks per day. Overconsumption of alcohol increases the risk of cancer, liver disease and alcoholism.

F. Y. I. *A simple way to eat for health and reduce your risk of heart disease, cancer and hypertension is the so-called "5-A-Day For Better Health" program. It's recommended that all Americans consume a variety of fruits and vegetables daily in these categories:*

1. Eat five servings of fruits and vegetables every day.

2. Eat a least one vitamin A-rich selection every day: e.g., apricots, cantaloupe, carrots, spinach, squash.

3. Eat a least one vitamin C-rich selection every day: e.g., orange, grapefruit, tomato juice, broccoli.

4. Eat a least one high-fiber selection every day: e.g., figs, prunes, dried peas, beans.

5. Eat cabbage family (cruciferous) vegetables several times per week: e.g., broccoli, cabbage, cauliflower.

Source: U.S. Department of Agriculture

BUILDING BLOCKS OF NUTRITION

The ancient Egyptians built the pyramids from the bottom up. The U.S. government recommends that modern Americans apply that same principle to their eating habits.

The Department of Agriculture recently issued a "Food Pyramid" that lays out the U.S. Dietary Guidelines in graphic form. You should eat more servings of foods listed at the base of the pyramid—breads, cereals, fruits and vegetables—and fewer servings of high-fat foods listed at the top (see illustration below).

The focus of the Food Pyramid is on the prevention of disease. The guidelines are based on the latest scientific research from organizations such as the National Institutes of Health, the American Heart Association and the American Diabetes Association. Scientific studies show that good nutritional habits can lower your risk of heart disease and some cancers.

Following are some ideas about how to build the pyramid principle into your everyday life.

• **Breakfast:** Don't neglect breakfast! It's your most important meal of the day. Eating breakfast helps you feel alert and can save you from mid-morning snack binges. Try these tips:

- *Instead of high-fat eggs, bacon and doughnuts, try cereal, low-fat yogurt or cottage cheese, or a bagel with a low-fat spread. Always try to include a piece of fruit.*

- *If it's hard to find time for a sit-down breakfast at home, you can eat fruit and a bagel in the car or on the bus. Or try getting to work a little earlier and eating a "brown-bag" breakfast.*

- *Experiment: If you don't like regular breakfast foods, try lunch or dinner food instead.*

- *If you're at a fast-food restaurant, order the pancakes instead of the high-fat croissant or biscuit sandwich.*

• **Lunch:** No matter where you eat lunch—your desk, the cafeteria, a restaurant—you can make it nutritious and enjoyable. A bonus: a lunch that's lower in fat will help you avoid mid-afternoon sluggishness. Here are a few suggestions:

- *Try packing a balanced brown-bag lunch: a vegetable like cut-up celery; a sandwich with turkey, chicken or tuna (hold the mayo!); a piece of fruit; fig bars or graham crackers. Or instead of the sandwich, bring leftovers from home.*

- *If you eat in the cafeteria, try the salad bar. Be sure not to load up your plate with hidden fats: salads made with mayonnaise; heavy dressings. Your cafeteria may also offer special "health plates."*

- *If you're eating out, try to select main dishes that are broiled or steamed instead of fried. Also try to include a vegetable side dish, or order a*

FAT
Use Sparingly

DAIRY
2 servings per day for adults

BEEF, PORK, POULTRY, FISH AND EGGS
2 to 3 servings at 2-3 ounces per serving.

FRUITS AND VEGETABLES
5 to 6 servings per day. Each serving equals 1/2 to 1 cup.

BREADS, CEREALS, GRAINS, PASTAS AND STARCHY VEGETABLES

PREVENTION

12

main-dish salad. Most fast-food restaurants now post nutritional information: some of it may surprise you.

- **Snacks:** Snacking can help you meet your daily dietary requirements and gives you a satisfying pick-me-up in the mid-morning or late afternoon. Try these ideas:

  - raisins or other dried fruit

  - low-fat crackers, pretzels or popcorn

  - fresh fruit or vegetables; canned fruit packed in water

  - unsweetened cereal; bagels

  - Low-calorie puddings

  If you make regular trips to the vending machine, find out what's in the food you select. Is it high in fat? Sodium?

- **Dinner:** With today's busy schedules, it's often hard to plan ahead for dinner. Try doing your planning during your trips to the grocery store, stocking up on fruits, vegetables, pasta, rice, whole-grain breads and lean meats to have on hand for quick meal preparation. Also consider these suggestions:

  - To cut down on fat, broil meats instead of frying them. Be sure to trim all visible fat from meat before cooking.

  - Try to round out your daily recommended servings of fruits and vegetables (at least five servings). Microwave cooking is great for vegetables: it helps to preserve nutrients.

  - Be aware of hidden fat in cheeses, sauces, gravies, dressings and nuts.

- **A word about beverages:** It's a healthy idea to drink six to eight 8-ounce glasses of water daily, to aid in digestion and weight control. Also, try to moderate your consumption of caffeine, alcohol and sugary drinks. Fruit juice, sparkling water and non-caffeinated tea make good substitutes.

- **Write it down:** You can become more aware of your eating habits by writing down what you eat, just as you keep track of your spending habits by recording checks in your checkbook. A food diary can help you see at a glance if you're eating for good health.

RESOURCES:

Eat for Life, Catherine Woteki and Paul Thomas, eds. Washington, D.C.: National Academy Press, 1992.

USDA's Food Pyramid Guide
USDA Home and Garden Bulletin No. 252
Consumer Information Center
Dept. 159-Y
Pueblo, CO 81009
$1 per copy
Make check payable to "Superintendent of Documents."

WEIGHT MANAGEMENT: KEEPING IT SIMPLE

Losing weight—and keeping it off—can benefit your health as well as your appearance, helping to lower cholesterol and blood pressure and reducing the risk of stroke, heart disease and diabetes.

Many people try to lose weight through crash diets or programs that promise quick weight loss. The fact is, there's no really effective quick-fix diet plan. Instead, we need to focus on successful weight management, which involves three key concepts:

Avoid Crash Dieting

Permanent weight loss doesn't result from drastic methods: losing weight rapidly through crash diets usually leads to a gradual return of body fat within six months. For many people, weight loss and gain becomes a repeated cycle. Research suggests that this practice, called "yo-yo dieting," increases the risk of coronary heart disease, especially among men. To keep weight off permanently, experts recommend that you lose no more than two pounds per week.

For most people, weight gain can be traced to two main factors: 1) food choices that are too high in fat; and 2) lack of physical activity. In most cases, successful weight management comes from making small changes in your everyday eating and activity patterns.

Make A Long-Term Commitment

A successful weight-management program involves long-term behavior change that aims for a gradual reduction in body fat rather than body weight. Inches lost is a better measure than pounds lost, since it indicates that you are increasing your lean body mass (muscle) and reducing your total percentage of body fat. *Approaching weight loss as a gradual process instead of a crash program is a safer and more effective way to take control of unwanted fat.*

Have A Positive Imagination

Someone once said: "When it comes down to willpower vs. imagination, imagination always wins." Most people blame their weight problems on a lack of willpower, when in fact they may simply need to do some positive thinking. During any behavior change, it's important to focus on the positive benefits of your change (e.g., more energy, better appearance, improved health) and not on what you're giving up. It's also important to believe that you can and will change. Treat any progress toward your goal as a mini-victory. And don't get discouraged if your progress levels off for a time—it happens. Stick to your plan and focus on the positive.

IDEAS THAT WORK:

Here are some simple strategies for taking charge of your weight.

• **Eat less fat.** A diet that gets 30 percen—or fewer— of its calories from fat can help you avoid a variety of health problems. Forty percent is the average for American diets.

Several studies now show that a low-fat diet will help you shed excess pounds, too. Suggestions for reducing fat in your diet:

- Substitute high-fat/high-calorie foods with low-fat/lower-calorie alternatives.

For example:

- Watch your snacking. Try to select low-fat foods. Read food labels carefully. Select snacks from vending machines such as low-fat yogurt, fig bars, raisins and popcorn. Try fresh fruit and cut-up vegetables instead of pastries.

- Be prepared. Watch how you prepare and cook your foods. Trim excess fat from meats. Remove skin from poultry. Try to broil or bake rather than fry meat selections.

WEIGHT MANAGEMENT: KEEPING IT SIMPLE

PREVENTION

14

- Undress. A low-fat baked potato or salad "dressed-up" can quickly become a fat/calorie nightmare. Try low-fat yogurt instead of sour cream and cheeses on your baked potato. Try vinegar and oil or low-fat dressings instead of regular high-fat salad dressings.

• **Increase your daily physical activity.** Physical activity is one of the cornerstones of weight management. If you've been inactive, adding physical activity to your life will increase your success in losing fat and maintaining ideal weight—as well as improving

HIGH-FAT CHOICE	SUBSTITUTE
Whole milk	Skim milk
Pork sausage	Low-fat ham
Fried potatoes	Baked potato
Baked beans	Green beans
Breast of chicken with skin	Skinless breast of chicken
Doughnuts	Bagel
Marbled beef	Lean beef

your overall health. Regular physical activity includes exercise such as walking, cycling and swimming—of 20 to 60 minutes duration, three to five time a week—combined with everyday activities such as manual labor, gardening and other household chores. Exercise not only burns calories and fat during your activity, but also keeps your body burning calories for hours after you stop. Exercise also increases your lean body mass (muscle), which, unlike fat, burns calories while the body is at rest.

Note: *If you're over age 40 and have been inactive, or have a medical condition such as high blood pressure, heart disease, diabetes or joint problems, consult your doctor before starting a weight-loss and exercise program.*

Your exercise program doesn't need to be strenuous for you to realize significant weight reduction. For example, moderate, sustained activity such as 40 minutes of walking five days a week can produce significant weight loss within 12 weeks. See Walking, p. 8.

• **Eat smaller portions and more often.** Instead of having three large meals, break up your daily diet into five to seven smaller meals helps your body use calories more efficiently.

• **Look at the mirror, not the scale.** As fat is converted into lean body mass (which is more dense and therefore heavier than fat) your weight may actually go up for a while. That's OK. You're becoming trimmer, healthier.

• **Keep a diary.** In a log, write down your eating habits: when you eat, what you eat, who's with you, your mood (e.g., bored, nervous, hurried, insecure). This helps you identify common eating triggers that most likely are not related to hunger, but are habits you've learned over the years: for example, snacking while watching TV.

• **Drink plenty of water.** Ironically, if you drink sufficient water, your body won't try to retain so much of it.

RESOURCES:

The Duke University Medical Center Book of Diet and Fitness, by Michael Hamilton, et al. New York: Fawcett Columbine, 1991.

The Fast Food Guide, by Michael F. Jacobson and Sarah Fritscher, eds. New York: Workman Publishers, 1991.

SHARPEN YOUR STRESS MANAGEMENT SKILLS

Stress is your body's response to what it understands to be a threat. Stress begins as a physical reaction, which makes you behave and think in ways that will help you handle the threat. In itself, stress is not unhealthy; in fact, it is one of the many responses your body uses to help you survive.

Things that you perceive as threats are called stressors. In general, physical threats create stress in all of us. But threats don't have to involve physical harm to be stressful. The threat could be to your self-esteem, as when somebody verbally abuses you, but you may have the same feeling as if you were being physically attacked.

Stressors vary from person to person. Something that you consider threatening might not bother others at all.

It's important to keep stress from becoming too overwhelming and a regular part of your life. That's why it's useful to develop a "suitcase" of different skills to help you cope with or rise above the various kinds of stress that may appear in your life. The following ideas can be used along with other strategies to help you manage stress in a positive way.

IDEAS THAT WORK:

• **Set your course.** Take the time to draw up a life plan for the next three to five years. In a notebook, list the answers to the following basic questions. Every month, take out your list. How are you doing? Do you need to change your plan? Try to be honest with your answers.

- *What do you want your life to become?*

- *Who are the people you want to share it with?*

- *What do you need to do to achieve your goals?*

- *What resources do you need: people, money,*

information, time?

- *Where does your job fit into your plan?*

• **Develop your other life departments.** There's more to life than just your job, and thus there are many opportunities outside of work for achieving personal growth and increasing life satisfaction. People who are most effective in dealing with personal stress are those who not only have a clear picture of their goals, but also are well-balanced in other parts of their lives.

Try this little quiz. At this time in your life, how would you rate the following areas as either helping or hurting your life goals and satisfaction, or not making any difference (neutral)?

LIFE DEPARTMENT	HELPS	HURTS	NEUTRAL
Physical	❑	❑	❑
Mental/Emotional	❑	❑	❑
Knowledge	❑	❑	❑
Career	❑	❑	❑
Family	❑	❑	❑
Social/Community	❑	❑	❑
Financial	❑	❑	❑
Spiritual	❑	❑	❑

How did you do? Look at the departments that you rated as hurting or not making any difference to your life goals: you may need to spend more time and energy in developing these areas of your life. If you have more departments that help your life goals, you're generally able to manage stress better and "bounce back" sooner.

• **Be prepared.** When you expect to encounter something stressful, have the knowledge, skills or tools that you need ready to go. For

PREVENTION

16

example, if you know you will have added responsibilities at work or at home, identify available resources that can help you balance these added pressures. Prepare family members and coworkers for the changes—ask them for their help and understanding.

- **Describe the stressful situation.** If you have time, write down the problem. Break it down into parts: how do you react to and act on a specific situation? This will help you see the whole picture and how your behavior affects other parts of your life.

- **Gather support through family and friends.** To deal positively with stress, it's important to have a close network of friends and family to talk and share feelings with. A strong social network can improve your overall outlook on life and its problems, make you aware of other perspectives and make you feel that you're not alone in making important decisions.

- **Learn to communicate better.** Many stress problems happen because we fail to communicate. Learn to become an active listener. Listen to another person's message without "coloring" it with your own biases and preconceived ideas. Also, try to express yourself—your feelings, thoughts, concerns—rather than striving to impress others by "winning" every conversation.

- **Stay healthy.** By practicing basic life-skills such as being physically active, eating right, controlling your weight, moderating your use of alcohol, avoiding drugs and tobacco, and learning to relax, you can go a long way in helping cope with stressful times.

- **Avoid alcohol or drug dependence.** Using drugs or alcohol is a common way for some people to cope with stress. If you think you have a substance abuse problem, please get professional help.

- **Learn to use relaxation techniques.** Practice calming techniques such as meditation, exercise or prayer to help bring stress under control.

- **Look stress right in the eye.** Accept that a certain amount of unmanageable stress will naturally and certainly happen. Resolve to deal with it. Try to change your attitude toward it, rather than running away or ignoring it.

- **Seek professional help if necessary.** If you feel you just can't cope by yourself, get help from a mental health professional. Good resources include your company or union employee assistance program (if offered), your minister or rabbi, and community mental health centers.

RESOURCES:

Mind as Healer, Mind as Slayer, by Kenneth R. Pelletier. New York: Dell Publishing, 1992.

The Seven Habits of Highly Effective People, by Stephen R. Covey. New York: Simon & Schuster, 1989.

15 Quick Fixes To Reduce Stress

A major key to stress control is being able to manage day-to-day stressors before they reduce your personal effectiveness. The following self-care skills can be used to help you avoid overload and reduce tension in your everyday life. When the cause of your stress is more serious, quick fixes are not enough. Refer to Resources on p. 124 for additional assistance.

IDEAS THAT WORK:

- **Pace yourself.** Pace your workflow—on and off the job—whenever you can, by staying organized, setting realistic timelines and having needed resources available before you begin any project. Try to set aside 20 percent of your time for unplanned events or problems.

- **Avoid overloading on caffeine.** Coffee, tea and cola drinks are stimulants that increase your heart rate and can make you more irritable. Try caffeine-free beverages instead.

- **Use your imagination to relax.** When you're feeling tense, find a space where you can sit quietly for 10 to 15 minutes. Try this visualization exercise:

   - *Close your eyes.*

   - *Breathe normally.*

   - *Visualize yourself as a burlap bag full of sand, full of tension.*

   - *Your feet are the bottom corners of the bag.*

   - *The corners suddenly burst open, and the sand begins to run out.*

   - *Feel the sand run out of your feet, and all the tension that you feel run out, too.*

   - *Completely empty the bag of all the sand…all the tension.*

   - *Resume your normal activity.*

- **Control your breathing to relax.** Most meditation exercises use breathing techniques to help relax the body and the mind. Try this simple relaxation technique:

   - *Find a private spot where you can be quiet for 10 to 15 minutes.*

   - *Sit erect, with your hands in your lap.*

   - *Close your eyes.*

   - *Inhale deeply, hold your breath for five seconds and exhale slowly.*

   - *Sit quietly, concentrating on your breathing. Breathe through your nose.*

   - *On every exhale, say the word "calm."*

   - *With every exhale, feel your mind becoming more still.*

   - *Don't fight other thoughts or distractions; let them come…let them go.*

   - *Just concentrate on your breathing.*

   - *After 10 to 15 minutes, open your eyes. Remain seated for two to three minutes.*

   - *Resume your normal activity.*

- **Tense, then relax.** Progressive relaxation is a popular relaxation technique that has been used for years. The idea is first to tense, then to relax, specific muscle groups in a regular order. Try this technique when you begin to get tense:

   - *If possible, find a private, quiet room.*

   - *Lie on the floor. (If that's not possible, sit comfortably in an armchair.)*

   - *Loosen any tight clothing: belt, necktie, collar. Remove your shoes.*

   - *Close your eyes and breathe normally.*

   - *For each muscle group, tense the muscles for six*

seconds, then relax. Repeat three times before going to the next group of muscles.

- The sequence: feet, calves, thighs, buttocks, shoulders (bring shoulders to ears if sitting, up off the floor if lying down), hands, forehead, jaw (make a face, stick out your tongue).

- Reverse sequence.

- **Walk it off.** A simple 20- to 30-minute walk has been shown to reduce muscular tension as much as some tranquilizers.

- **Stretch it out.** Simple stretching exercises are an effective way to reduce built-up tension in the neck, shoulders and back.

- **Have a good belly laugh.** Some experts call a good laugh "inner jogging." Keep a book of jokes or humorous short stories close by. If you begin to feel angry or tense, take a humor break.

- **Tune Up!** Playing classical or other selections can help you relax and concentrate. There are also a number of relaxation tapes that combine nature sounds or soothing music with self-suggestive instructions that either ask you to visualize a specific scene or teach you to relax specific muscle groups.

- **Keep a journal.** A popular and effective way to manage stress is to keep a daily journal. Journal writing allows you to note your feelings on a given day: problems, insights, solutions and outcomes. Many journal keepers find the exercise of journal writing a means of blowing off steam. Your journal can also be a record of personal growth.

- **Stop that thought!** When you have a stressful or negative thought, try this technique:

- Stop the thought in midstream. Actually say to yourself: "Stop!"

- Take a deep breath and exhale slowly.

- Mentally, take a step back...look at the situation objectively.

- Ask yourself: "Is my reaction (perception) overblown?"

- Then ask yourself: "What's a more positive, constructive way to approach this problem?"

- **Pray.** Many experts, have shown that prayer is a very effective calming technique, comparable to other relaxation and meditation techniques.

- **Game it.** Simple mental diversions such as puzzles and video and computer games can take the edge off seriousness, ease tension and even release a creative urge or two.

- **Book power.** Read a favorite book.

- **Doodle.** Remember when your first-grade teacher had you finger paint? Well, creative outlets also calm the soul. Have a few crayons on hand. Next time you get stuck on a problem, annoyed or tense, return to Ms. Smith's class and doodle for a few minutes.

RESOURCES:

The Relaxation Response, by Herbert Benson, M.D. New York: Avon Books, 1976.

You Don't Have to Go Home From Work Exhausted!, by Ann McGee-Cooper, Duane Trammell and Barbara Lau. Dallas: Bowen & Rogers, 1990.

Your local mental health agency. Check your phone directory under "Mental Health."

Your health care provider.

Empowerment, by Dennis Jaffe and Cynthia Scott. Los Altos, Calif.: Crisp Publications, 1991.

HEALTH SCREENINGS

Health screenings have become a major topic of debate in the health community. Prestigious organizations such as the National Academy of Sciences, the American Cancer Society and the U.S. Department of Health and Human Services all have recommended decreasing the frequency of many types of health screening tests. Although there is a tremendous benefit in the early detection of disease, periodic health screenings need to be used carefully especially among individuals at low risk and a young age. Not only is mass testing expensive, especially among low risk groups, but "negative" results can lead to further tests that have their own risks and usually are more expensive (see below).

Today, it is recommended that individuals have selective health screenings based on their age, sex and relative health risks (e.g., a family history of breast cancer). These periodic screenings take the place of the traditional "annual" checkup, which consists of a comprehensive battery of tests such as blood work, resting or exercise electrocardiogram (EKG), and chest X-ray.

The following are reasons for not having a comprehensive screening:

1) Many "preventive screening tests" do not guarantee that hidden diseases will be detected. The best method to determine if testing is necessary is through reported symptoms (e.g., chest pain on exertion, swollen glands or chronic fatigue).

2) Some "positive tests" may in fact be "false positive," which can lead to more expensive tests that may place you at greater risk.

3) You will save money. Comprehensive physical examinations can cost from $300 to $1,000 and, again, may have limited value in detecting hidden disease.

It is recommended that you have some tests on a periodic basis. The chart on the following page highlights some of the most common tests for the general population. Schedules are based on age or sex, and may take into consideration relative health risks, such as family history of disease. In some cases, screenings (blood pressure and cholesterol) are offered through health fairs, worksite health promotion programs or local not-for-profit health agencies (e.g., the American Heart Association and the American Cancer Society) at little or no cost to the public.

Note: Recommendations vary as to the frequency of testing. Talk to your doctor about what is best for you, based on your personal and family health history.

RESOURCES:

Common Screening Tests, by D.M. Eddy. Philadelphia: American College of Physicians, 1991; (215) 351-2626.

Guide to Clinical Preventive Services: An Assessment of the Effectiveness of 169 Interventions. Report of the U.S. Preventive Services Task Force. Baltimore: Williams and Wilkins, 1989.

COMMON HEALTH SCREENING TESTS: RECOMMENDED SCHEDULES

TEST	AGE			
	20–29	30–39	40–49	50 and over
Blood Pressure	• Every one to two years, unless part of a doctor visit for another purpose.			
Cholesterol/HDL	• Screening every five years from ages 36 to 70, after one test between ages 21 and 35 (unless results are elevated). See pp. 101 and 102.			
Pap Smear	• Once sexual activity begins or at age 21. If test is negative after three consecutive yearly tests, then repeat every three years at your doctor's discretion.			
Mammography			•Baseline mammogram may be recommended.	•Every year
Dental Exam	• Dental cleaning and exam recommended every 6 to 12 months. • X-rays are not recommended unless the patient has cavities or pain.			
Breast Exam By Physician			• Every year	• Every year
Breast Self-Exam	• Breast self-exam should be performed every month.			
Testicular Self-Exam	• Monthly examination after shower when scrotum is relaxed.			
Occult Blood (for rectal cancer)				• Every year
Prostate (digital exam)			• Every 2 years	• Every year
Sigmoidoscopy				• Every 3 to 5 years

IMMUNIZATIONS

RECOMMENDED IMMUNIZATION SCHEDULE FOR COMMON INFECTIOUS DISEASES		
Protection from:	**Abbreviation**	**Age**
Diphtheria, pertussis, tetanus	DPT	2 months 4 months 6 months 18 months
Polio	OPV (oral)	2 months 4 months 6 months (high-risk areas) 18 months 5 years
Bacterial meningitis	Hib	2, 4, 6 and 18 months**
Measles, mumps, rubella*	MMR	15 months
Measles		4 to 5 years of age
Tetanus/adult diphtheria	Td	5 years of age Every 10 years thereafter
Hepatitis B	HBV	All infants—at birth, 2 and 6 months. Individuals at high risk (e.g., health care workers).**
Influenza (yearly strain)	Influenza	Yearly for adults who are 65 or older, or who suffer from chronic conditions such as heart or lung disease or have impaired immunity.
Pneumonia	Pneumovac	One-time shot—for adults who are 65 or older, or who suffer from chronic conditions such as heart or lung disease or have impaired immunity.

* Women and teenagers of childbearing age should be tested for antibodies against rubella (German measles). Immunization should be done if no antibodies are found. Talk to your health care provider. ** Your physician may recommend alternative schedules based on vaccine used or age at first dose.

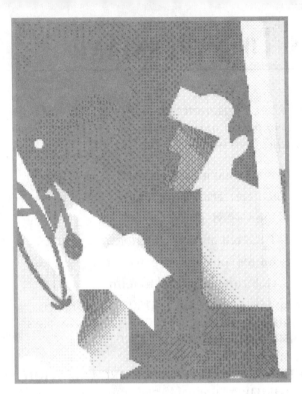

Understanding The Basics Of Medical Care

BY USING THIS SECTION YOU WILL:

• Learn common health care terms.

• Learn how to select a primary care physician.

• Learn how to talk to your doctor and what key questions to ask.

• Learn how to locate health information and resources to make better informed decisions.

As employers, insurance companies and the government try to manage exploding health care costs, new terms are becoming part of the health care vocabulary. Here are some of the most common terms.

TERMS TO WORK WITH:

- **CAPITATION:** A set dollar limit that you or your employer pays a health maintenance organization (HMO), regardless of how much you use the HMO's services, or a flat fee paid to a health care provider.

- **CASE MANAGEMENT:** A service that assigns a health professional (usually a nurse) to monitor, with the physician and the hospital, the care plans of individuals who require extensive medical treatment. The case manager's primary responsibility is to make sure that the individual receives the most appropriate and reasonable care.

- **COINSURANCE:** The amount patients are required to pay through their insurance plan for reasonable medical expenses after a deductible has been paid (also referred to as a "copayment" in some plans). Usually insurance plans require a 20 percent contribution by the patient, with 80 percent paid by the employer or insurance company.

- **COPAYMENT:** A flat fee that is paid by the patient on a per visit basis. For example, HMOs may require a $5 to $10 "copay" for each office visit.

- **DEDUCTIBLE:** A minimum payment made by an individual and/or family before the company or insurance carrier begins to pay for medical expenses.

Example: *John Wright broke his leg during a softball game. His company has a deductible of $150, coinsurance of 80/20 percent, and an out-of-pocket maximum of $2,500. His entire medical bill was $850.*

John's total medical bill	$850
John's personal charges are:	
- John's deductible	$150
- Total bill minus deductible	$700
- John's coinsurance percentage	×20%
- Coinsurance charge to John	$140

John is required to pay: $150 (deductible) + $140 (coinsurance) = $290. His company pays $850 (total medical bill) – $290 (John's charges) = $560.

- **HEALTH MAINTENANCE ORGANIZATION (HMO):** A "pre-paid" or "capitated" medical system in which members receive medical services for *one monthly fee*, regardless of the severity of the problem or number of visits. HMOs are usually either a Staff Model or an Independent Practice Association (IPA).

In the Staff Model, dedicated clinics and staff are located within the community and treat subscribers only and/or employees of the HMO. IPA physicians are contracted to provide services out of their own offices, not a centralized facility, and can treat non-HMO patients.

- **INDEMNITY HEALTH PLAN OR "FEE-FOR-SERVICE" PLANS:** Under this type of plan, the employer or insurance company pays a percentage (usually 80 percent) of the cost of each medical service received by the eligible patient. The patient's contribution is called coinsurance. Indemnity plans usually require the employee to pay a certain amount for medical expenses (a deductible) before the employer or insurance company begins to contribute.

Health Care Terms To Understand

- **MANAGED CARE:** A medical care delivery system that manages health care and costs through a variety of services designed to provide quality care appropriate to patients' needs. Most managed care programs involve a network of primary care physicians (HMOs and PPOs), specialists and hospitals.

- **MAXIMUM DOLLAR LIMIT:** The maximum amount of dollars the employer or insurance company will pay within a specified period of time. Maximum dollar limits can be for a lifetime ($ 1 million) or for a year, or can be illness-specific, such as for psychiatric care or cancer treatment.

- **OUT-OF-POCKET MAXIMUM:** The maximum amount that a patient is required to pay through coinsurance before the employer or insurance company pays 100 percent of reasonable medical expenses. Common in fee-for-service plans.

- **POINT-OF-SERVICE (POS):** A managed care system in which participants' care is managed by their primary care physician, much like an HMO. In a POS plan, participants can choose their network providers for a moderate copayment. However, participants have the flexibility in using non-network providers. They need to meet a deductible and pay a larger copayment.

- **PRE-CERTIFICATION OR PRE-ADMISSION REVIEW:** A process that requires patients with certain medical conditions to contact a health professional before medical reimbursement is approved.

- **PREFERRED PROVIDER ORGANIZATION (PPO):** A network of physicians and hospitals that agree to give discounts to companies when employees use their services.

- **PRIMARY CARE PHYSICIAN (PCP):** A physician who is responsible for monitoring and treating your general health needs, such as performing periodic health screenings and immunizations, and treating common medical problems. Typical PCPs are internists (who treat adults only), family physicians (who treat adults, children and infants) and pediatricians (who treat infants and children up to age 18.) See p. 26.

- **NURSE PRACTITIONER:** A Registered Nurse (RN) with advanced training that prepares him/her under a physician's supervision, to provide routine checkups and to help manage minor, acute and chronic health problems.

- **PHYSICIAN'S ASSISTANT:** A health care professional with medical training that allows him/her under a physician's supervision to provide routine health maintence checkups and to manage minor, acute and chronic health problems.

- **REASONABLE AND CUSTOMARY FEES:** The approved amount an insurance carrier or company will pay for a specific medical or dental procedure. Charges above this amount are the responsibility of the individual.

- **SECOND OPINION PROGRAMS:** A cost management process that requires patients to seek the counsel and opinion of a second physician in certain situations: for specific medical procedures that are elective; when other accepted options for treatment exist; when the diagnosis is still in question; or when hospitalization or surgery is recommended.

- **SPECIALIST:** A physician trained and certified to treat a specific body system, such as a cardiologist (problems of the heart), gynecologist (woman's reproductive system) or dermatologist (skin problems).

THE BASICS

25

FINDING DR. RIGHT

Medicine has changed a lot over the last 40 years. The house call has been all but eliminated. It has been replaced by urgent care centers, 24-hour clinics and the long office visit. Most Americans don't have a "Dr. Welby" who treats them from cradle to grave. Instead, more than 50 percent of Americans meet their doctor for the first time during a medical need or emergency. This meeting in a crisis is not the best way to build a relationship, especially as you are trusting someone with your own or your family's care and well-being. An important first step in being a good medical consumer is finding a doctor you can relate to and trust.

IDEAS THAT WORK:

• **Find a Primary Care Physician (PCP).** Your primary care physician is responsible for your "primary care"—caring for your general health needs, such as performing periodic health screenings and immunizations, and treating common problems that don't require a specialist. Approximately 70 to 80 percent of all medical problems can be treated by a well-trained PCP.

It's to your advantage to find a PCP. Because your PCP knows you and the two of you have developed a good relationship, he or she can help you avoid unnecessary tests and procedures that can be expensive and possibly place you at greater risk. When a medical problem is more serious, your PCP may refer you to a specialist, but is still involved in your total care plan.

• **Select your Primary Care Physician according to your needs.** Shop for a doctor who can meet most of your medical needs and those of your family. As a first choice, a doctor certified in family practice or as a

general practitioner may be able to meet your needs and provide a cohesive care plan that includes lifestyle management. However, your family may need more than one PCP. For example, in a young family of three, the husband may have an internist, the wife an obstetrician-gynecologist and the child a pediatrician. If this is the case, physician selection should be based on the qualities listed below.

Look for a PCP who:

❏ Is a person you feel confident about and respect.

❏ Has good communication skills: he or she is an active listener and takes time to talk and explain things.

❏ Believes in prevention and provides information to assist you.

❏ Chooses tests and procedures carefully, and prescribes medication carefully.

❏ Is willing to accept what is called "Reasonable and Customary Payment."

❏ Has a reasonable waiting time for appointments, e.g., less than five days.

❏ Can and is willing to be contacted by phone.

❏ Has established after-work office hour scheduling arrangements.

• **Use your network.** Ask friends, family members and coworkers to suggest doctors. Find out the reasons why they like a specific doctor or why they dislike others. Do not automatically rule out someone based on a negative comment. For example, a doctor may have a poor "bedside manner," but be excellent in his or her specialty.

• **Ask the pros.** Contact your local medical society, teaching hospital (talk to the chief resident for recommendations) or your preferred hospital. Whenever possible, talk to nurses, who usually have excellent views of a doctor's professional reputation, skills and attitude toward patients. If a specialist is needed, ask your PCP for at least two recommendations.

- **Call a physician line.** A number of "Physician Referral Services" are currently available. When you call an advertised phone number, a consultant will help match you to a doctor based on your health needs, location and personality preferences. Beware. Though these services can provide you with a list of doctors or even schedule an appointment for you, they usually are paid for and run on the behalf of the doctors who join the service.

- **Is he or she certified?** Some studies suggest that doctors who are "board certified" may provide more appropriate care. When a physician is board certified, it means that he or she has passed a national standardized test of competency.

- **Refer to your insurance plan.** If you belong to a Health Maintenance Organization (HMO), you may select or be assigned a PCP or be referred to a doctor, depending on your medical need. If you do not like your assigned physician's performance, request another doctor.

  If your company health plan is part of a Preferred Provider Organization (PPO), you may want to select a PCP from a "preferred list" of doctors. You will receive discounts if your doctor is part of the PPO. Use the suggestions above to help you select a PCP from the list.

- **How's the office staff?** How are you treated on the phone and in the office? A friendly, responsive office staff usually reflects a doctor with a similiar manner.

- **How long do you need to wait?** How are appointments scheduled: for example, four patients per hour or 10? Ask about the usual waiting time. Look at how many people are waiting in the reception area; this can give you a pretty good hint on office scheduling procedures.

THE BASICS

27

F.Y.I.

Remember, your Primary Care Physician should be viewed as your partner in health. By selecting a qualified doctor with whom you can communicate and share decisions, you can get better medical care, help avoid unnecessary medical procedures, lower your out-of-pocket expenses and stay healthier.

Another option for your preventive health care needs is using the services of a nurse practitioner or physician assistant. Talk to your PCP if this option is available.

THE BASICS

The visit to the doctor's office has been a source of jokes for many comedians and TV shows. Many Americans are frustrated by the long waits, the impersonal way patients are herded between examining rooms, the short time allowed for them to talk to their doctor, questionable tests, and of course the high costs. The medical establishment is not insensitive to these issues. In fact, surveys indicate that doctors want to spend more time with their patients. By following the strategies below, you can improve the quality of the office visit for yourself, the doctor and other patients, too!

IDEAS THAT WORK:

• **Question the need.** Estimates show that approximately 25 percent of all visits to the doctor are not needed. Either there is nothing the doctor can do—as in the case of uncomplicated colds—or other health professionals can be used, as in the case of routine screenings for blood pressure or cholesterol. The first question you should ask is: "Do I need to see my doctor, or do I have other options such as applying self-care?"

• **Be prepared.** If you are going to your doctor with a new problem, it is important to provide the right information. Don't be embarrassed or scared. Try to share your thoughts and observations on the cause of your problem or other medical concerns (past or present). This will help your doctor narrow down the diagnosis and develop a treatment plan. If possible, write down the answers to the following questions before your visit:

❑ **What is your primary problem?** Be specific by listing your key symptoms; for example: I have had stomach cramps and diarrhea.

❑ **When did your problem begin?** Try to give the exact time. If you cannot pinpoint the exact date that a symptom appeared, try to remember the general period that you began to notice you weren't feeling well.

❑ **What do you think may have caused the problem?** Did you eat some unusual food? Do any family members or coworkers have similar symptoms?

❑ **Know your family history.** Is there a history of such diseases as heart disease, high blood pressure, diabetes and breast cancer among your immediate family: parents, grandparents, brothers or sisters?

❑ **What have you done to try to relieve the problem?** Have you used any medications? What kind? What happened?

❑ **Did you have this problem before?** When? What happened?

❑ **What makes the problem worse?** List what activities, medications, foods or other situations makes your problem more serious.

❑ **Are you allergic to any medications?** If yes, what are they?

• **Answer questions as best you can.** Your doctor may ask you detailed questions by body system (e.g., symptoms related to your skin, head, eyes, ears, throat, etc.) to see if there are any patterns to your problem. You will also be asked about your family life, emotional health, potential job-related exposures, and general health behaviors such as alcohol consumption, drug use, tobacco use, exercise habits and sexual activity. Though these questions are personal, it is important to be direct and honest with your responses.

• **Cooperate during the checkup.** When your doctor has finished his or her questions, you usually receive a focused physical examination. Once again, it is important to answer directly any questions that you may be asked. You have the right to question or refuse any recommendations. State your concern. Listen to your doctor's reasons.

• Diagnostic tests. Doctors often use diagnostic tests to better determine either the cause of an illness or how serious it is. Ask questions about the benefits (e.g., will it change my treatment if I have this test?), risks and costs.

• Use the INFORMED Process. *If your problem is complex and requires intensive testing and treatment, it's to your advantage to use a more formal way of deciding on your care plan. The INFORMED Process, explained in detail on pp. 34 through 37, can help you and your doctor in considering your treatment options.*

• Follow through with treatment. To avoid more serious and expensive procedures and treatments, it is important to understand and follow the treatment plan you have agreed to. Many recurring medical problems are caused by patients' taking shortcuts in treatment. A common cause is not following through on medications: taking the wrong dosage; stopping medication too early; and not adhering to the daily schedule. Another cause is over-medication. A common belief is, "If one pill is good, then two must be better." Medications are of value only when taken as directed. If you are concerned about your medication, discuss it with your doctor.

Finally, don't ignore suggestions that seem too simple, such as drinking plenty of fluids, getting bed rest, eating a balanced diet, stopping smoking, exercising or losing weight. These recommendations are just as sound as other high-tech medical advice, and in fact are often the best medicine you'll ever give yourself.

F.Y.I.

As outlined above, it's important to follow through with your care plan as directed by your doctor. Most of us tend to forget details over time. Therefore, it's recommended that you <u>write</u> <u>down</u> *what your doctor tells you. Here is a summary:*
• *Write your care plan on the same sheet of paper where you listed your symptoms.*
• *Write down the diagnosis.*
• *Write down your treatment plan: medications (see Medication Use, p. 47), nutritional needs, activity restrictions, special exercises and other specifics.*
• *Have your doctor identify any possible medication side effects (use Medication Use Record, p. 123).*
• *List what warning signs (e.g., infection, high fever) require further medical evaluation.*
• *Finally, don't be afraid to ask your doctor to clarify a point if you don't understand.*

Most patients don't question their doctor. They may feel they have no right to challenge someone who's had at least 11 years of formal education, or they feel embarrassed or "stupid," especially when the problem is serious. Instead of giving up control, most experts believe, it's important for you to become **more involved** in your care plan. *The more information you have, the more active you can become in making decisions concerning your health.* Remember that the first skill in being a good medical consumer is asking the right questions. But don't expect to get all your questions answered completely all the time. Medicine is a complex science, and **uncertainty** is a fact of life.

Basic Communication Tips

The following are some basic guidelines for improving your communication skills with your doctor. *When **more complex medical procedures** (e.g., surgery, hospitalization, diagnostic tests) are recommended, it's suggested that you use the **INFORMED Medical Decision-Making Process** and Worksheet (See pp. 34 through 37).*

- **Write down your questions.** Organize your questions and concerns before you visit your doctor.

- **Don't feel intimidated or "stupid."** Ask questions when you don't understand an explanation. Ask your doctor and other health professionals to simplify their response by stating it in nontechnical terms.

- **When tests are prescribed, question their value and need.** For example: "If I have this test, how will it change the outcome of my problem?"

- **When a treatment is prescribed, ask what other options are available.** For each option, have your doctor explain the risks, benefits and total expense.

- **When medication is prescribed, ask about signs of adverse reactions.** Be sure you understand the recommended dosage and schedule.

F.Y.I.

THE SECOND OPINION:
In cases of elective surgery, or when you aren't sure about your treatment plan, it makes sense to get a second opinion. Check with your insurance company or your primary care physician to find a specialist.

*Your insurance carrier may require you to contact them before you proceed with certain procedures. This **pre-certification process** helps ensure that your surgery or treatment plan is the right one for your needs. If a second opinion is required, your insurance carrier will usually pay the bill.*

*Talk to your doctor and hospital before an elective medical procedure is done to make sure they will accept what is considered a **"Reasonable and Customary"** cost for the procedure. If they agree, you won't have to pay anything above what your insurance agrees to pay. If not, you will be required to pay the difference between what your insurance provides and the cost of the procedure.*

FACT-FINDING: LOCATING MEDICAL RESOURCES

To become an informed consumer of health and medical services, it's important to have adequate information and resources concerning your health problem. Information enables you to ask your doctor the right questions about such topics as available treatment options and their relative risks, benefits and costs.

IDEAS THAT WORK:

Here are some suggestions for researching your medical or health problem:

• **Start with your Primary Care Physician.** Sit down with your PCP and have him or her help you address the questions that are listed on the *INFORMED Worksheet* on pp. 34 through 37. If your doctor doesn't have the time, ask if a staff member can help you. See if your PCP has any pamphlets, videos or other educational material that describes your condition and is targeted to the layperson.

• **Get a second opinion.** If you question your doctor's recommendations, consult another doctor for a second opinion. In fact, your insurance plan may require it, especially in the case of elective surgery.

• **Patient Counseling Services.** Your company, in cooperation with its insurance carrier or an independent consultant, may offer telephone medical counseling services that do the fact-finding for you. This type of a service is *not* a diagnostic service, nor does it recommend treatment; rather, it helps coach you to ask your doctor the right questions regarding your health problem.

• **Tele-Medicine Services.** Many local hospitals and HMOs provide educational services you can access through your telephone. An automated system allows you to select audiotapes that explain a health condition.

• **Go to a college or a medical school library.** If you live close to a medical school or college,

try to access their library. A medical library is more comprehensive than a college library, and will give you more disease-specific information.

• **On-line Computer Services.** If you have a home computer and subscribe to an on-line service (e.g., *America Online and Prodigy*), find out if they have on-line health and medical files you can access. Many on-line services also have electronic bulletin boards that allow members to post and respond to questions left within the network. But be sure to question information and advice that promise quick cures and sound too good to be true.

• **Support Groups.** Many support groups (e.g., multiple sclerosis, AIDS, breast cancer) have their own resources you can access. Check with your local hospital, health department, not-for-profit agencies and on-line services for support groups near you.

• **Governmental Agencies.** The U.S. Government, through the National Institutes of Health, have various publications and some hotlines (e.g., cancer, AIDS) that provide educational assistance to individuals. You can also contact NIH regarding any clinical trials of experimental treatments that may be in effect and find out what admission criteria is required to be part of these government-financed studies.

• **Not-For-Profit Groups.** Organizations such as the American Academy of Family Physicians, the American Cancer Society, the March of Dimes, the American Heart Association, the National Multiple Sclerosis Society, the Asthma Foundation, the American Diabetes Association and the American Red Cross have their own educational materials and programs you can request.

RESOURCES:

Refer to pp. 124 through 126 for organizations and other resources.

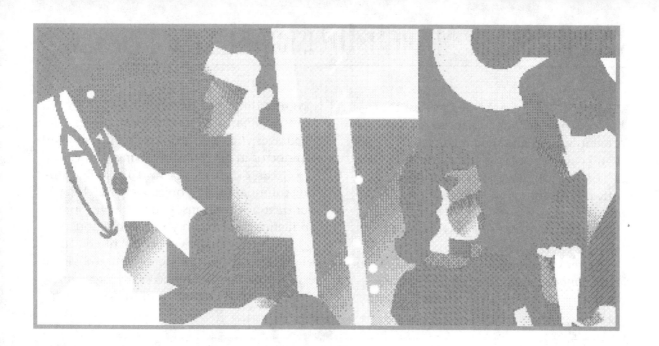

The INFORMED Medical Decision-Making Process

By Using This Section You Will:

• Learn the INFORMED Medical Decision-Making Process.

• Learn how to be an active partner with your doctor regarding treatment decisions.

• Learn how to avoid hospitalization and reduce your medical costs.

• Learn about your rights as a patient and what documents you can't live without.

D E C I S I O N - M A K I N G

INFORMED is an eight-step process that allows you and your doctor to explore treatment options and their relative risks, benefits and costs when faced with a major medical decision (e.g., surgery, hospitalization, diagnostic testing and/or another treatment option).

The advantages of using this decision-making process include:

• **Better Communication:** INFORMED provides a *uniform process* that requires you and your doctor to communicate about key questions regarding your treatment.

• **Participation:** The eight-step process encourages you to be an active participant with your doctor in decisions involving your care.

• **Greater Confidence And Trust:** By gathering information and objectively weighing your treatment options, you will have more confidence and trust in your treatment plan.

• **Improved Quality:** You will receive medical care that is appropriate for your individual needs. By decreasing unneccessary procedures, you will probably reduce your total care costs.

THE INFORMED DECISION-MAKING PROCESS™

The primary goal of INFORMED is to help you become a more active participant in decisions regarding your medical care. You can help remember the INFORMED process by memorizing the decision-making sequence below:

Input: What is my problem? What are my doctor's recommendations: further diagnostic tests, medications, surgery, hospitalization?

Need: Why do I need treatment? What happens if I do nothing? What do I expect from my doctor?

Fact-Finding: Aside from my attending physician, do I need further information and resources to make a better informed decision? Do I need to get a second opinion? (See p. 30.) Fact-finding includes addressing the following areas:

Options: Do other options exist for my problem? What are they? Can they be ranked from least intensive (e.g., "do nothing") to most intensive (e.g., surgery)?

Risks/Benefits: For each option, what risks exist (e.g., infection, permanent disability, other complications, death)? Also, what are the benefits of each option (e.g., complete recovery, lower cost, avoiding surgery, avoiding hospitalization)? How do the benefits of each option meet my needs: e.g., complete cure vs. minor disability or discomfort?

Management: For each option, will there be a need to manage my problem after my primary treatment? For example, will I need to be on medication(s) for an extended period of time? Will I have to eliminate or reduce certain activities including my work? Will I need rehabilitation? What can I do to help prevent my problem from happening again?

Expense: What is the total cost of each option? Total cost includes: medical costs, time off from work, lost wages, emotional distress, loss of independence, disfigurement due to scarring, etc.

Decision: After weighing each available option with my doctor, which one seems the most appropriate for my situation?

INFORMED WORKSHEET

PLEASE PHOTOCOPY

Whenever you or a family member is faced with a medical problem that requires more intensive treatment (e.g., comprehensive diagnostic tests, surgery, hospitalization), make a copy of this worksheet and take it with you when you visit your doctor. Ask your doctor to help you complete the worksheet.

It is important to remember that there's always a degree of *uncertainty* in medical treatment. Though this worksheet can help you and your doctor "walk" through your treatment options, you may desire further information and additional fact-finding may be necessary.

Step One: Input

Q1) Does your doctor know what your medical problem (official diagnosis) is?
Yes _____ (Go to Q2) No _____ (Go to Q4)

Q2) What is the the name of your problem (diagnosis)?

_____

_____

_____

Q3) What is your doctor recommending to treat your problem? What's involved?

_____

_____

_____

_____

Q4) If your diagnosis is not known, what are the possible explanations for your symptoms? What further tests is your doctor recommending?

_____

_____

_____

_____

Step Two: Need

Q5) Why do you need to have your problem treated or a certain test done?

_____

_____

_____

_____

Q6) What would happen if you chose not to have a treatment or test done?

_____

_____

_____

_____

Q7) What are your expectations of your doctor? How realistic are your needs?

_____

_____

_____

_____

Step Three: Fact Finding

Q8) Besides your doctor, where else can you find out more about your problem (e.g., publications, other health professionals, organizations, support groups)?

_____

_____

_____

Step Four: Options

Q9) What options may be appropriate for treating your problem?
List them in the appropriate boxes within the chart on p. 37.

DECISION-MAKING

35

D E C I S I O N - M A K I N G

Step Five: Risks/Benefits

Q10) For each identified option, what are the potential risks (e.g., infection, disability, death, future surgery)?

Q11) For each identified option, what are the potential benefits (e.g., no surgery, no hospitalization, no scarring, less cost)?

List both risks and benefits under each option on the chart.

Step Six: Management

Q12) For each option, will any short-term and/or long-term management be required (e.g., medication, rehabilitation, housing needs, nursing needs, nutritional needs, activity or job restrictions) for your problem?

List these considerations under each option within the chart on p. 37.

Step Seven: Expense

Q13) For each option, what are the estimated total costs? If applicable, include costs of tests, surgery, medications, hospitalization, and doctor's fees. Also try to estimate the indirect costs such as lost wages, lost time, emotional costs, disability and loss of independence, disfigurement due to surgery, etc.

List your estimated costs under each option on the chart.

Q14) What procedures and tests are covered by your insurance carrier?

Q15) Does your insurance carrier require you to contact them before an elective procedure is approved (pre-admission review)?

Q16) Does your doctor(s) and hospital accept what your insurance company considers to be reasonable and customary fees?

Step Eight: Decision

Q17) After evaluating your available options with your doctor, which one seems to be the best option for you?

Q18) Are there any additional questions you need to have answered?

Q19) What is the next step to implement your care plan?

INFORMED Option Comparison Chart

	OPTION ONE	OPTION TWO	OPTION THREE
CHOICE	Do nothing (Watchful Waiting **)		
RISKS			
BENEFITS			
MANAGEMENT			
EXPENSE			
DECISION	☐	☐	☐

** "Doing Nothing" involves no medical or surgical treatment. You continue observing (watchful waiting) your symptoms for improvement, worsening or no change over a specified period of time. Based on your observations, future treatment may be advised by your doctor.

DECISION-MAKING

37

DECISION-MAKING

Forty-four cents of every health care dollar is spent on hospitalization and its related tests and procedures. Because hospitalization is the most expensive part of health care, everyone is trying to reduce unneccessary hospital visits and find alternatives (e.g., home care, ambulatory surgical centers) that provide quality care at a lesser cost.

Avoiding unnecessary hospitalization should be a major goal of any wise consumer of medical services. Hospitalization has its own potential risks (e.g., infection, complications during surgery or diagnostic testing, adverse reactions to medications and inactivity) even in the best institutions. Be sure to question the need for hospitalization when it's recommended. *See the INFORMED Worksheet starting on p 35.*

Of course there are legitimate reasons why hospitalization is justified (e.g., emergency trauma, complicated surgical or treatment procedures). However, even in these situations, you should be active in the decision-making process whenever possible.

The following are examples of key questions that you should discuss with your doctor when hospitalization is recommended.

Questions Regarding Hospitalization And Surgery:

- **Outpatient vs. hospitalization?** If surgery or hospitalization is recommended, find out if there are any other options, like medications and outpatient surgery services, to treat your condition.
- **Explore all options whenever possible.** If options exist, ask your doctor about their benefits, risks and costs. See *INFORMED* on p. 34.
- **Question the *total* cost.** Besides the monetary costs of a specific treatment, ask your doctor about the potential physical and

emotional costs of a specific treatment plan, e.g., post-operative depression and disfigurement due to surgery. *See INFORMED on p. 34.*

- **Pre-plan your surgery and treatment plan.** When surgery or other intensive treatments (e.g., chemotherapy) are recommended, become aware of what to expect during the recovery or treatment phase.

Key questions:
- ❏ *How much pain should I expect from my incision or procedure?*
- ❏ *How long does it normally take to completely recover from this kind of surgery?*
- ❏ *What are the risks of disability because of my surgery, e.g., nerve damage, limited mobility?*
- ❏ *What will my treatment be after my surgery?*
- ❏ *What signs should I look for that indicate that the treatment is working?*
- ❏ *What are the possible complications of my treatment?*
- ❏ *What signs should I look for that indicate I may have a problem?*
- ❏ *What problems should I call you about?*
- ❏ *How long will I be out of work?*
- ❏ *Are there certain activities that I shouldn't participate in for a while? If yes, how long should I wait?*

- **If a surgical specialist is recommended, don't be afraid to ask questions, such as:**
- ❏ *Are you board certified?*
- ❏ *How many surgeries similar to mine have you done?*
- ❏ *What is your success rate?*
- ❏ *Who will assist you?*
- ❏ *What is his or her experience?*
- ❏ *Will he or she actually do the surgery and you assist?*

It's estimated that up to 99 percent of all hospital bills have at least one error—usually an overcharge. The larger the bill and the longer the hospital stay, the greater the chance is that there will be errors in your bill. This does not mean that your health care provider is intentionally charging you for services not given. It simply means that mistakes happen, especially when many people are involved in your care, and your medical condition calls for more intensive treatment.

With the high cost of medical care, it's important that you pay only for those services that have been rendered. If you don't, your company or insurance company will pay more (which increases everyone's premiums), and your own out-of-pocket costs will increase.

IDEAS THAT WORK:

Here are some ways to reduce your hospital bills and protect your pocketbook:

- **Reasonable and Customary? Not!** Before agreeing to a medical procedure, make sure your doctor will accept what your insurance company will pay. This is called a reasonable and customary (R&C) charge. If your doctor charges more than the R&C, you will be stuck with the difference. When in doubt, always check with your insurance carrier before approving an elective treatment.

- **Is pre-certification required?** For many elective medical procedures, your insurance carrier requires that you contact them before your treatment proceeds. Through this process, called *pre-certification review*, your carrier helps you decide if the treatment is required or other options are available. Failure to use the pre-certification process can land you with the entire medical bill or

a higher deductible. Read your health benefit material carefully.

- **Outpatient services?** Be sure to ask your doctor if a certain procedure (e.g., minor surgery) can be done on an outpatient basis instead of in the hospital. If hospitalization is required, avoid weekend admissions, since many diagnostic services are limited. Also, find out if any X-rays, lab tests or blood work can be done on an outpatient basis before you're admitted.

- **Check your deductions and out-of-pocket maximums.** Errors can occur when your insurance company fails to calculate your deductible correctly or charges you beyond your out-of-pocket maximum. Make sure you understand your health benefit plan. Carefully review your insurance statement for possible mistakes.

- **The meter is running.** Once you're admitted to the hospital the charges begin. In reviewing your bill make sure your admission and discharge dates are correct. As with hotels, you may be charged a fee for being discharged after a certain time of the day. Refuse this charge if the hospital delayed your departure.

- **Log it!** Keep a detailed record of what tests, drugs and other services you receive on a day-to-day basis, or have a family member do it for you. Don't be shy about asking medical personnel what a certain dressing or drug is if you don't know.

- **Bring your own medications.** The $5 charge for an aspirin is normally a big shock to the first-time hospital patient. Bring your own medications (e.g., aspirin, ibuprofen) with you, as well as prescription drugs you cur-

DECISION-MAKING

DECISION-MAKING

rently use. Before using any drug, check with your doctor to make sure that the drug is needed or if it may interfere with your current treatment.

- **Itemize!** Always ask for an itemized list of all services performed instead of a cost summary. Compare the list to your log and identify any services that you believe were not given. Report these questionable charges to your health insurance plan.

- **Stick to your guns.** If you feel you have been overcharged and are getting nowhere with the hospital billing department, work with your insurance company. Also, contact your state agency that regulates hospital finances: they may be able to help you in reducing your charges. Remember, though, it's important to have documentation (e.g., a log) to support your case.

RESOURCES:

Your insurance carrier.

Your company benefit department.

Your state regulatory agency for hospital financing.

PATIENT RIGHTS

To be an informed medical consumer, it's important for you to understand your rights and responsibilities, and to respect the fact that medical personnel must conform to their own professional code of ethics and practices. The American Hospital Association (AHA) has developed a document entitled *Your Rights as a Hospital Patient* to help patients become aware of their rights and the hospital's responsibilities in treatment. Although written for hospital patients, most of these principles are important for all patients—hospitalized or not.

According to the American Hospital Association:

• You have the right to considerate and respectful care.

• You have the right to be well-informed about your illness, possible treatments and likely outcome and to discuss this information with your doctor. You have the right to know the names and roles of people treating you.

• You have the right to consent to or refuse a treatment, as permitted by law, throughout your hospital stay. If you refuse a recommended treatment, you will receive other needed and available care.

• You have the right to have an advance directive, such as a living will or health care proxy. These documents express your choices about your future care or name someone to decide if you cannot speak for yourself. If you have a written advance directive, you should provide a copy to the hospital, your family, and your doctor.

• You have the right to privacy. The hospital, your doctor, and others caring for you will protect your privacy as much as possible.

• You have the right to expect that treatment records are confidential unless you have given permission to release information or reporting is required by law. When the hospital releases records to others, such as insurers, it emphasizes that the records are confidential.

• You have the right to review your medical records and to have the information explained, except when restricted by law.

• You have the right to expect that the hospital will give you necessary health services to the best of its ability. Treatment, referral, or transfer may be recommended. If transfer is recommended or requested, you will be informed of risks, benefits, and alternatives. You will not be transferred until the other institution agrees to accept you.

• You have the right to know if this hospital has relationships with outside parties that may influence your treatment and care. These relationships may be with educational institutions, other health care providers, or insurers.

• You have the right to consent or decline to take part in research affecting your care. If you choose not to take part, you will receive the most effective care the hospital otherwise provides.

• You have the right to be told of realistic care alternatives when hospital care is no longer appropriate.

• You have the right to know about hospital rules that affect you and your treatment and about charges and payment methods. You have the right to know about hospital resources, such as patient representatives or ethics committees, that can help you resolve problems and questions about your hospital stay and care.

Used with permission, the American Hospital Association, 1992.

DECISION-MAKING

ADVANCE DIRECTIVES: STATING YOUR WISHES

DECISION-MAKING

Although medical technology can keep patients alive indefinitely, many people do not want *heroic measures* to be taken if there is minimal chance of recovery. They don't wish to lead a life of such compromised quality, or to be an emotional or financial burden on their families. Yet many people are unable to communicate their wishes at the time when a decision must be made. Health care professionals, bound by a duty to protect life, often are caught in a dilemma.

To address this problem, health care advocacy groups have lobbied in most states for the right of citizens to specify in advance—through legal documents called "advance directives." These documents are prepared before you are faced with a life-threatening condition or major medical procedure.

IDEAS THAT WORK:

Most advance directives are either *a living will* or a *durable power of attorney for health care.*

- **Living Will.** A formal document that is signed, dated and witnessed by two people who are not involved in your health care and are not future heirs to your estate. A living will states what kind of life support and heroic measures you wish to receive if you're not able to make those decisions at the time and your condition has been listed as terminal. Living wills can also specify what other medical procedures can be performed. It's usually recommended that a lawyer review your document, though it's not required.
- **Durable Power of Attorney for Health Care.** A formal document that is signed, dated and witnessed, naming another person to make medical decisions for you in the event you are unable to make decisions on your own. A lawyer is not required to write a durable power of attorney for health care.

Things To Keep In Mind:

- **Legality?** Most states legally recognize advance directive documents; each state has its own requirements. Refer to Resources below.
- **Which one?** Depending on the state you live in, one document or both may be recommended. Advance directives usually can be combined, specifying not only life support limitations, but also the type of care you wish to receive if you're unable to make decisions on your own.
- **Second thoughts?** *You can cancel or change your specifications at any time.* You can also change your orders to your doctor by oral communication.
- **No directives, what then?** If you have provided no advance directives and your illness prevents you from making any care decisions, your family, doctor and hospital are responsible for your treatment plan. Sometimes a judge may be needed if there is disagreement about treatment options.

RESOURCES:

Choice in Dying
200 Varick St.
New York, NY 10014
(212) 366-5540

Your local Area Agency on Aging. Call the Eldercare Locator Service at (800) 677-1116 for the AAA nearest you.

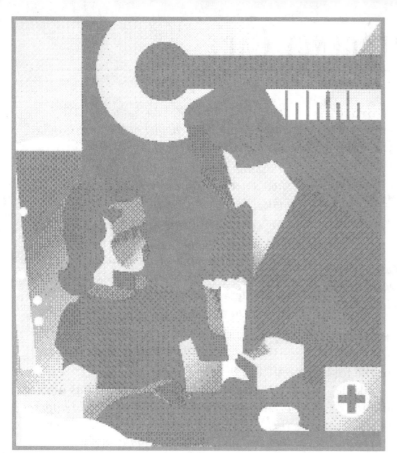

Treating Common Medical Problems

By Using This Section You Will:

• Learn about the 45 common medical problems that account for most doctor visits.

• Learn how to determine if a certain problem needs medical attention.

• Learn how to apply HomeCare for medical problems that don't need a doctor's treatment.

• Learn how to reduce your out-of-pocket medical expenses by reducing unnecessary doctor visits.

It's estimated that up to one third of Americans visit an emergency room every year. For the majority of cases, the emergency room is the wrong treatment choice because the medical problem doesn't require urgent care. Many conditions can be treated by your primary care physician or at home, resulting in less wasted time and emotional distress, and considerable cost savings.

Not only is the emergency room an expensive option, an overload of nonurgent cases can also slow down the response of medical staff to more serious problems.

It's important to be aware of conditions that do need emergency care. You should seek immediate medical attention for any of the following conditions by calling 911 (if available) or the operator (dial 0) for an ambulance or emergency response team:

- *Possible signs of heart attack. Signs may include severe pain in the middle of chest, pain in jaw or upper back, numbness or pain that spreads to arms (especially left arm), shortness of breath and cold sweats.*

- *Possible signs of stroke. Signs may include sudden fainting, dizziness, slurred speech, changes in vision, stupor, disorientation and/or marked weakness on one side of the face or one or more extremities on the same side of the body.*

- *Unconsciousness. You are unable to awaken the person.*

- *Extreme difficulty breathing. This may indicate a severe allergic reaction or an asthma attack.*

- *The person is not breathing or has no pulse. If you are alone and a phone is nearby, call for help first, then apply CPR. If you're not alone, send one person to call for help immedi-ately and apply CPR. You can learn CPR through your local chapter of the American Red Cross or American Heart Association.*

- *Possible spinal cord injury. The person should not move or be moved if there is an injury to the neck or back.*

- *Severe bleeding. Bleeding cannot be stopped after you have applied direct pressure for 10 minutes and you have no assistance. If you have assistance, drive the person to the closest urgent care center while your companion applies direct pressure to wound.*

• Other conditions that require urgent care (call the emergency room or your primary care physician first):

- *An infant under 3 months old has a fever of 101 degrees F or higher—(rectal temperature). This condition could indicate a serious infection and needs immediate attention.*

- *Severe vomiting or diarrhea, especially in infants.*

- *Poisoning. First, try to locate the toxic agent. Read the label and call your poison control center (find the number in phone directory and keep it by all phones). Follow their instructions carefully. See p. 46, Poisoning.*

- *A serious injury. Possible broken bone(s), a head injury (without loss of consciousness), serious burns.*

- *Severe pain. Unexplained pain that doesn't go away or gets worse.*

Whether you're traveling in the United States or abroad, if you're really sick it's important to get medical attention right away. Your hotel may have a doctor on call. If you're in a foreign country, the nearest U.S. embassy will have a list of doctors in the area and will assist you in times of medical emergency.

According to the American Medical Association, you may need immediate medical attention if you have any of the following symptoms:

- *Fever over 101 degrees F for two days or longer*
- *Chills with shaking*
- *Stiff neck*
- *Diarrhea, vomiting and abdominal pain for more than two days*
- *Persistent heart palpitations or chest pains*
- *Coma or seizures*
- *Prolonged or severe weakness*
- *Prolonged asthma*
- *Extensive bleeding from the mouth, nose, ears or rectum*
- *Poisoning, bites by venomous animals*
- *Bone fractures*

If your medical problem is very serious, don't take the time to contact the embassy to call a doctor. Call a taxi or an ambulance to take you to a hospital emergency room.

IDEAS THAT WORK:

The following is a checklist for travelers who have medical conditions that may require attention away from home.

- **Consider a medical exam before leaving.** Be sure to have an examination if you plan to be out of the country for an extended period of time.
- **Are you covered?** Be sure to check with your company or insurance carrier to make sure your health insurance will cover you at your destination.
- **Bring your medicine.** Carry enough medication to last the entire trip plus extra for unexpected delays returning home. Don't forget medication for headaches, colds and allergies when appropriate.
- **Carry medications in their original containers.** Keep them in your carry-on luggage to avoid losing them.
- **Medical records.** Take a copy of your personal medical records with you.
- **Identify yourself.** Wear a Medic Alert bracelet if you have a medical condition that warrants it.
- **See clearly.** Take extra glasses, contact lenses and lens cleaning solution.
- **Authorize.** If you are leaving children at home, make sure you sign an authorization for medical treatment and leave it with your children's caretakers before you leave.

RESOURCES:

Medic Alert, Turlock, Calif.: (209) 668-3333

International Association for Medical Assistance to Travelers, Lewiston, N.Y.: (716) 754-4883

AirEvac: (800) 421-6111

SELF-CARE

45

Nearly 1.7 million poisonings occur in the home each year. Most poisonings occur when someone swallows a poisonous substance, but they also may result from exposure to a gas or absorption of a substance through the skin. The best prevention against poisoning? Taking the time to poison-proof your home—especially if you have young children—and knowing what steps to take if you think someone in your household has been poisoned.

IF YOU THINK SOMEONE HAS BEEN POISONED, DO THE FOLLOWING:

If the person is unconscious:

1. Immediately call 911 or the emergency room (keep phone number by all phones). Apply emergency resuscitation if there's no breathing or pulse.

If the person is conscious:

1. Call the poison control center immediately (keep phone number by all phones), even if you're not sure a poisoning has occurred. *If you have the poison in hand, do not follow instructions on the label unless you're unable to reach the poison control center.*

2. Answer the questions from the poison control center as best you can: e.g., victim's age, the name of the poison, when it was taken, whether the person has vomited.

3. Follow the instructions that are given to you.

- If the person has swallowed an acid, an alkali or a petroleum product, do not induce vomiting: this can cause more harm. You'll probably be instructed to first have the person drink milk to dilute acid or alkali products. Water should be used for petroleum products.

- If the above substances were not involved, you may be instructed to induce vomiting either by putting a finger to the back of the throat (this stimulates the gag reflex) or by giving syrup of ipecac. *Make sure you have syrup of ipecac in your home medicine cabinet. It can be purchased at your local pharmacy.*

4. Follow instructions for further medical care.

F . Y . I .

TO POISON-PROOF YOUR HOME, FOLLOW THESE SUGGESTIONS:

• *Keep things out of sight, up high and locked up. Take precautions with medicines, household cleaners, anything that contains alcohol, and houseplants.*

• *Watch medications. Be aware that child-resistant caps are not childproof—they just slow kids down.*

• *Use original containers. Never place poisonous liquids in other containers; they can be mistaken for something else.*

• *Keep your garage tidy. Keep gasoline, pesticides, paint products and antifreeze beyond the reach of young children. Use as directed.*

• *Make sure you keep syrup of ipecac available if there are children in the home.*

Medications, both over-the-counter and prescription drugs, need to be used wisely. Treat medications with respect by following the recommendations listed below.

IDEAS THAT WORK:

• Use the following checklist and your Medication Use Record on p. 123, when a drug has been prescribed. Ask your physician or pharmacist the following questions:

❑ *Why has this drug been prescribed?*

❑ *What are its possible side effects?*

❑ *Will it react with other drugs that I am taking?*

❑ *How long will I need to take this drug?*

❑ *What time of the day should I schedule my dose?*

❑ *If side effects occur, what should I do?*

❑ *What is the proper dosage?*

❑ *Should I take it on an empty stomach?*

❑ *Should I avoid alcohol or other foods or drinks?*

❑ *How will I know if the drug is working?*

❑ *Can this drug be substituted with a generic brand?*

❑ *How should this drug be stored?*

❑ *Are refills allowed?*

• Does the medication need to be reduced? Older adults metabolize drugs differently, and medications may remain in their bodies for a longer time. Therefore, they may need less than the usual adult dose.

• Beware of overmedication, or interaction with other drugs you may be taking.

• Medication by mail? If you need a drug for a long-term chronic condition, consider buying it from a mail-order drug company, for a savings of up to 50 percent. Contact your local or state pharmacy board or insurance company to locate suppliers. Your supplier should maintain a computerized medication file for each customer and provide a toll-free phone number for questions. Be sure to contact your insurance company concerning their coverage requirements.

F.Y.I.

KEEP THESE POINTS IN MIND CONCERNING SAFE MEDICATION USE

• *Know the name of the drug(s) you are taking. Know how often you are to take a prescribed or over-the-counter (OTC) medication and the proper dosage.*

• *Know how to take a drug properly: e.g., with water, on an empty stomach, etc.*

• *Know what drugs (prescription and over-the-counter medications) you're currently taking that should not be taken with this medication.*

• *Understand the side effects of this drug(s).*

• *Don't share your prescription drugs with another person or borrow someone else's.*

• *Don't change your dosage without first consulting your doctor.*

• *If possible, have all your prescribed medications come from one pharmacy or chain so that one source will have a record of all your medications. This will help minimize potential adverse drug interactions.*

The following list is provided to assist you and your family in stocking your medicine chest. It includes basic items for the treatment and relief of common medical problems. Before you proceed, take note of these recommendations:

- Discard any over-the-counter or prescription medications that have passed their expiration date.

- Never use another family member's prescription medication.

- Any drug can be harmful; read product information carefully and follow recommended dosages and schedules.

- Make sure all bottles are closed properly. Young children should be trained to stay out of the medicine cabinet—or better yet, lock the cabinet. Never leave any drug within the reach of small children.

RECOMMENDED SUPPLY CHECKLIST:

❑ Thermometer. Include rectal thermometer if household has young children.

❑ Blood pressure cuff (sphygmomanometer) and stethoscope if someone in your household has blood pressure problems.

❑ Aspirin, acetaminophen or ibuprofen. For fever, minor aches and pains, and headache;

F.Y.I.

Bringing a personal pharmacy to your place of work is not recommended. But because the majority of businesses have no occupational health nurse or infirmary to treat health problems, it is a good idea to have the following supplies stored in your desk, work station, locker or car glove compartment in case a need arises:

- *Aspirin, acetaminophen or ibuprofen for headache, fever or minor aches and pains*

- *Tissues*

- *An assortment of adhesive bandages for minor cuts*

- *Anti-bacterial soap to help clean minor cuts and other wounds*

- *Eye drops for minor eye irritations*

- *Saline solution for contact lenses, extra contact case, and possibly an extra pair of glasses*

- *Extra supply of tampons or feminine pads*

- *A list of relevant medical numbers, such as those of your primary care physician, local hospital, and your company medical clinic if you have one.*

In case of a job-related injury, be sure to understand your company's policy on reporting injuries.

aspirin or ibuprofen for reducing inflammation; ibuprofen for menstrual cramps.

❏ Antacid or sodium bicarbonate. For treating upset stomach.

❏ Antihistamines. For treating minor allergies such as hay fever, cold symptoms and some insect bites.

❏ Adhesive bandages, assorted sizes

❏ Gauze pads

❏ Disposable latex gloves

❏ Cotton balls and swabs

❏ Elastic bandage

❏ Scissors

❏ Tweezers

❏ Safety pins

❏ Toenail clippers

❏ Eye drops. To help with dry or itchy eyes.

❏ Hydrocortisone. For the treatment of skin rashes and itching.

❏ Petroleum jelly. For diaper rash or "jock itch."

❏ Pectin substance (e.g., *Kaopectate*). For controlling diarrhea.

❏ Syrup of ipecac. To induce vomiting upon poisoning. (Be sure you know when to use.)

❏ Antifungal powder or spray. To treat fungal infections such as athlete's foot.

❏ Sunblock or sunscreen (SPF 15). To prevent sunburn.

❏ Water-soluble lubricant (K-Y Jelly). For vaginal dryness.

❏ Zinc oxide preparation. To prevent sunburn.

❏ Dental floss. To prevent buildup of plaque on teeth.

POPULAR OVER-THE-COUNTER MEDICATIONS

DRUG/BENEFITS	COMMON BRANDS	POSSIBLE RISKS/DRAWBACKS
ASPIRIN • Relieves mild to moderate muscle pain • Anti-inflammatory agent • Relieves tension headaches • Relieves arthritis pain • Reduces fever	*Bayer, Anacin, Maximum Strength Anacin, Maximum Strength Bayer, Bufferin, Alka-Seltzer, Regular Strength Ecotrim, Empirin, Aspergum*	• Stomach upset, stomach and duodenal ulcers, or gastrointestinal bleeding • Reye's syndrome in children and teens • Increased risk to woman or fetus in last trimester of pregnancy • Aspirin poisoning
ACETAMINOPHEN • Relieves mild to moderate muscle pain • Relieves headaches • Does not irritate stomach • Recommended for children and teens with fever to prevent Reye's syndrome	*Regular* and *Extra Strength Tylenol, Excedrin P.M., Liquiprin, Anacin 3, Datril*	• Liver damage in excessive amounts (greater than 5,000 mg) • Alcoholics at greater risk for liver damage • Does not reduce inflammation • No effect on arthritis
IBUPROFEN • Relieves muscle pain and soreness • Reduces menstrual pain • Relieves headaches • Useful in treating strains and sprains • Reduces fever • Relieves arthritis	*Advil, CoAdvil, Medipren, Motrin-IB, Nuprin, Pamprin-IB, Alka-Setlzer Plus*	• Stomach upset, stomach and duodenal ulcers, or gastrointestinal bleeding • Potential kidney damage to people with kidney disease
COLD PREPARATIONS • Relieve cold symptoms: fever, muscle aches, nasal congestion. Dry mucus.	*Contac, Coricidan, Dristan, Triaminic*	• Drowsiness • Agitation • Possible upset stomach
ANTIHISTAMINES • Relieve and treat allergy symptoms • Relieve cold symptoms • Relieve itching • May be used for insect bites	*Chlor-Trimeton, Benadryl, Allerest, Sinutab*	• Drowsiness • Agitation • Nosebleeds • Difficulty wearing contact lenses • Difficulty urinating • Impaired functioning, i.e., operating machinery, driving
NOSE DROPS AND SPRAYS • Relieve congestion and runny nose	*Afrin, Contac, Dristan, Neo-Synephrine*	• After prolonged use, symptoms can become worse because nasal lining becomes dry and irritated, causing even more swelling. • Agitation and/or rapid heart rate
COUGH PREPARATIONS • Expectorant preparations loosen mucus • Suppressant preparations reduce the cough reflex	*2/G, Robitussin, Romilar, Cheracol-D, Robitussin-DM, Vicks Formula 44*	• Drowsiness • Constipation
HYDROCORTISONE CREAMS • Relieve itching and rashes from poison ivy, poison oak and insect bites	*CaldeCort, Cortaid, Dermolate, Bactine, Lanacort*	• Long-term use (more than two weeks) can lead to skin damage
LAXATIVES • Increase bulk to stool by drawing in water • Stimulate digestive tract (e.g. Ex-Lax)	*Effer-Syllium, Metamucil, Milk of Magnesia,* Bulk laxatives that contain psyllium. *Ex-Lax (stimulant)*	• Diarrhea • Dehydration with extreme cases of diarrhea
ANTI-DIARRHEAL • Thicken the stool or slow bowel • Relieve severe cramping	*Kaopectate, Metamucil Imodium A-D*	• No significant side effects • Nausea and sedation

This section is designed to help you determine if your medical problem needs the attention of a doctor. *When your medical problem does not require a doctor, you are referred to the HomeCare column on the right-hand side of the page.* Each HomeCare column has special picture boxes (icons) that suggest a certain order of treatment. For example, rest, medication and fluids may be recommended. Try the treatment in the order presented. *However, first be sure that your problem does not require medical attention by checking the section titled "Consult Your Doctor If."*

What Do The Self-Care Icons Mean?

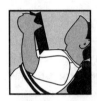

REST: When this icon is shown, it will recommend that you change or limit your overall activity level. *Bed rest usually will not be necessary.*

FLUIDS: When this icon is shown, it will recommend that you consume adequate levels of fluids to prevent dehydration, especially when a fever or diarrhea is present, or that you avoid certain drinks such as alcohol. Fluids also keep mucus more liquid and help you avoid secondary infections such as bronchitis. In most cases, water is the first choice, but it lacks needed minerals that may be depleted from your body because of illness. Therefore, fruit juices, electrolyte drinks (e.g., *Gatorade*) or caffeine-free carbonated drinks may also be recommended.

MEDICATION: When this icon is shown, specific over-the-counter medications will be recommended. It is important to keep the following points in mind:

- Use the specified medication as directed by the manufacturer. Read the instructions on the side panel carefully.

- Do not over-medicate. Don't use more than the directed dosage and recommended schedule.

- If you have a pre-existing health problem, such as hypertension or prostate enlargement, refer to the warning message on the label. If your problem is identified, do not use the medication without consulting your physician.

• Because of the risk of Reye's syndrome, do not use aspirin for children or teenagers who have symptoms of influenza (respiratory flu) or chicken pox. Use acetaminophen, either liquid (for infants and young children) or tablets, to treat fever and muscle aches.

NUTRITION: When this icon is shown, it will recommend either special meals, depending on your problem, or a balanced diet. When you have a fever, it is important to consume enough calories to maintain your strength and make up for calories burned because of increased body temperature.

51

HEAT/COLD: When this icon is shown, it will recommend that you apply either heat or cold to the injured area.

HEAT is used in therapy to bring blood and nutrients to an injured area. Hot compresses, heat packs and whirlpool baths help relax muscles that are sore and tense. Heat is not recommended when there is swelling and inflammation of a joint, especially within the first 48 to 72 hours after injury. Heat treatment will increase the swelling, bleeding and pain in the injured area.

COLD is used in cases of tissue swelling and inflammation. Cold temperatures constrict blood vessels, thereby slowing blood flow to the injured area, and reduce pain and discomfort. Commercial ice packs or ice cubes in a plastic bag are common ways to apply cold to an injured area. Another method is freezing styrofoam cups filled with water and peeling the top away when needed. Ice cups can be used when a joint such as an ankle or elbow needs to be massaged because of tendonitis. Ice therapy should be applied in intervals of 20 minutes on and 20 minutes off. *Be careful of frostbite: white skin and numbness.*

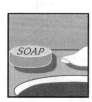

CLEAN: When this icon is shown, it will recommend ways to clean an injury such as a cut or abrasion, or an area of the body exposed to chemicals or other external irritants such as poison ivy. In most cases, plain soap and water will be recommended over alcohol and other antiseptic preparations.

COVER: When this icon is shown, it will recommend ways to bandage or cover a wound or injury. In some situations, the wound should not be covered unless there's an increased risk of infection, or pieces of clothing or other objects would rub and irritate the wound. Not covering the injury allows more oxygen to reach the wound, which speeds the healing process and decreases the risk of infection.

ACTIVITY: When this icon is shown, it will recommend either limiting physical activity to allow proper healing or special exercises to speed recovery.

OTHER: When this icon is shown, it will recommend additional methods for treating your problem at home.

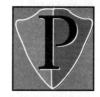

PREVENTION: When this icon is shown, it will recommend techniques that will help you prevent the problem from recurring.

Coughing is an automatic reaction to an irritation in the throat, breathing tubes or lungs. The irritation can be caused by dry air, tobacco smoke, allergies, a piece of food stuck in the airway or chemical fumes, or can be a reaction to a viral or bacterial infection.

If you have a viral infection, you may cough up yellow or white mucus. Green or rust-colored mucus often indicates a bacterial infection. Viral infections (e.g., colds and flu) need to run their course and usually don't need a doctor's attention. Bacterial infections, on the other hand, should be checked by your doctor, who will usually prescribe antibiotics as treatment. *Consult your doctor immediately if mucus is rust-colored, or is pink and frothy, and you have a fever of 102 degrees F or above. These symptoms may indicate pneumonia.*

Experts believe that you should not use cough suppressants if you have a *productive cough,* that is, you are coughing up mucus and other material. A productive cough is one way the body tries to rid itself of an infection.

With a *nonproductive* dry cough, you don't cough up any mucus. Throat lozenges, hard candies or over-the-counter cough suppressants that contain *dextromethorphan* may reduce the discomfort of nonproductive coughs and coughs caused by irritation in the back of the throat from post-nasal drip.

CONSULT YOUR DOCTOR IF:

- Your infant (under 3 months) has a cough.
- Your child has difficulty breathing, or is wheezing or breathing rapidly.
- You have a dry, nonproductive cough with no other symptoms, and it doesn't go away after one week.
- You cough up mucus that is rust-colored, or pink and frothy, and you have a fever of 102 degrees F or higher.
- You cough up mucus that is thick and green.
- Your cough hasn't gone away after you've recovered from a cold or flu.

HOMECARE

If physician referral is not recommended at this time, try the following self-care procedures:

- Drink plenty of fluids to help keep mucus more liquid and easier to cough up.
- Avoid caffeine drinks, e.g., coffee, soda and tea and alcohol, which increase urination.

- Use expectorants with care; try to loosen mucus through increased fluid intake first. Use expectorants as directed.
- If your cough is nonproductive, try a cough suppressant that contains dextromethorphan. Talk to your pharmacist.
- Try hard candy or throat lozenges to relieve an irritated throat.
- Antihistamines or decongestants may be tried to control post-nasal drip. Use as directed.

- Try a vaporizer to increase the humidity in your home, especially your bedroom.
- A hot shower can help thin mucus.
- Fill your bathroom sink with hot water and place a towel over your head. Form a tent over the sink and breathe in the steam for 10 minutes. Repeat as needed.

- If you smoke, try to quit.

*Because of the risk of Reye's syndrome, aspirin should not be given to or used by children or teenagers who have or are suspected of having flu or chicken pox. Use acetaminophen.

SELF-CARE

54

A sore throat can result from a number of factors, such as dry air, smoking (including passive smoking), allergies, air pollution, or a viral or bacterial infection. Mild throat irritation is common in people who sleep with their mouths open, which causes the throat to become dry and scratchy, or who have postnasal drip.

Viral infections such as influenza and colds are common causes of sore throat. A more severe sore throat occurs with mononucleosis. "Mono" is a viral infection common among *adolescents and young adults. Besides a sore throat, symptoms of mononucleosis include extreme fatigue and swollen glands.* It is important to remember that a viral sore throat *cannot* be treated with antibiotics.

Sore throats also can be caused by bacteria, usually from the streptococcal strain. *"Strep throat" symptoms are usually limited to pain in the throat, while a sore throat caused by a virus usually has other associated symptoms such as a runny, congested nose, headache and cough.* These symptoms indicate a typical cold or influenza and rarely require a doctor's visit (See p. 60, Colds and Influenza.) On the other hand, a strep throat needs to be diagnosed by your doctor through a throat culture. Untreated, strep can lead to rheumatic fever (mostly in children) or inflammation of the kidneys. *Antibiotics are the treatment of choice for strep and **may** sometimes be prescribed for family members as a preventive measure.*

CONSULT YOUR DOCTOR IF:

- Throat is bright red, or pus or white spots are present on back of throat and symptoms are limited to the throat only.

- Sore throat is accompanied by fever of 102 degrees F or above and symptoms are limited to throat only.

- A mild sore throat lasts more than two weeks.

- You have difficulty breathing or swallowing, or your child displays excessive drooling.

HOMECARE

If physician referral is not recommended at this time, try the following self-care procedures:

- Viral infections need to run their course. Bed rest usually is not needed.

- Fluids will help relieve soreness. Try weak tea with honey and lemon to soothe the throat.

- Aspirin, ibuprofen or acetaminophen for fever.*
- Decongestants with or without antihistamines for runny nose.
- Cough drops to soothe a dry throat.

- Salt water gargles may ease soreness.
- Try a humidifier in your home, especially in bedrooms.
- A vaporizer can help also.

- If a household member has strep throat, your doctor may prescribe antibiotics for everyone else. Smokers are more prone to upper respiratory infections.

*Because of the risk of Reye's syndrome, aspirin should not be given to or used by children or teenagers who have or are suspected of having flu or chicken pox. Use acetaminophen.

Contrary to general belief, an elevated body temperature is not necessarily an indication of illness. Your body temperature changes throughout the day and night in response to stress, physical activity, hormonal changes and even as a reaction to spicy foods.

Most medical experts agree that "fever" is when body temperature measured with an oral (mouth) thermometer is higher than 100 degrees Fahrenheit. Fever in itself is not a disease, it's the body's defense against infection. Many bacterial and viral infections are destroyed by an increase in body temperature; fever is therefore a normal and welcome response. Fever in adults usually is not serious unless it occurs in combination with other symptoms such as stiff neck (possible meningitis), severe diarrhea or abdominal pains.

CONSULT YOUR DOCTOR IF:

- Adult or child: fever is combined with a stiff neck (difficulty touching chin to chest), confusion and lack of energy.

- Adult: fever of 104 to 105 degrees F has not been reduced after three days of HomeCare.

- Adult: fever lasts longer than five days.

- Infant **under 1 month** of age with a temperature of **100.4 degrees F or greater as measured by a** *rectal* **thermometer.**

- Infant from **1 to 3 months** of age with a **rectal** temperature of **101.4 degrees F or greater.**

- Infant **under 3 months** of age has a *rectal* temperature of **100.4 degrees F for more than 24 hours.**

- Child **3 months to 2 years** has a *rectal* temperature of **101.4 degrees** F for **more than three days** without other symptoms, or **fever increases,** or fever is accompanied by **other symptoms,** e.g., vomiting, diarrhea.

- Child **3 months to 2 years** who has a *rectal* temperature of **103 degrees F.**

- Child with fever show **signs of so-called "fever fits" (febrile seizures).** Children between 6 months and 4 years of age are at greatest risk. **Symptoms:** Fever of 104 to 105 degrees F; muscles stiffen throughout the entire body, eyes may roll, the child's head may jerk, hands and/or feet may tap, and loss of bowel and urine control may occur.

HOMECARE

If physician referral is not recommended at this time, try the following self-care procedures:

- Aspirin, ibuprofen or acetaminophen for reducing fever higher than 101 degrees F. Use as directed.*

- It's important to maintain fluid balance. Drink plenty of water. Other caffeine-free drinks like fruit juices or ginger ale can be used.

- Sponge the skin with lukewarm water (not cold water). Evaporation will have a cooling effect on skin and bring heat to surface.

- Limit your activity. Bed rest may be advisable in cases of high fever and other symptoms such as diarrhea.
- Limit a child's activity since it can increase temperature even more.

* Because of the risk of Reye's syndrome, aspirin should not be given to or used by children or teenagers who have or are suspected of having flu or chicken pox. Use acetaminophen.

Diarrhea is a common sign of a gastro-intestinal infection. Usually caused by a virus and sometimes by bacteria (e.g., food poisoning, poor drinking water), diarrhea is the body's way of clearing the infection from the intestine. Diarrhea usually is preceded by abdominal gas and cramping. When diarrhea is frequent or painful cramping occurs, an antimotility compound such as *Imodium A-D* is a useful over-the-counter preparation. Ask your doctor or pharmacist to recommend medication.

Other causes of diarrhea can be traced to medications such as antibiotics and drugs used to treat high blood pressure and arthritis. Nervous tension is another culprit that stimulates the digestive system.

CONSULT YOUR DOCTOR IF:

- Your diarrhea is black or bloody.

- You experience severe abdominal pain with diarrhea.

- You experience dehydration: increased thirst, dark yellow urine, limited urination and skin that may be wrinkled and have no tone.

- Diarrhea continues for more than 48 hours after following HomeCare procedures.

- You experience diarrhea that comes and goes for more than one week.

- You have begun to take a new medication.

- Your infant has any diarrhea episodes, is feeding poorly, appears listless and is less responsive to you.

HOMECARE

If physician referral is not recommended at this time, try the following self-care procedures:

- Slow down the activity of your digestive tract. Drink plenty of clear fluids: water, ginger ale or apple juice. **For infants, substitute milk with water or oral rehydration solutions such as OTC preparations *Pedialyte* and *Rice-a-lyte*.**

- OTC preparations that contain pectin (e.g., *Kaopectate*) solidify runny stools. Drink plenty of water with preparation.
- OTC preparations (antimotility compounds) such as *Imodium A-D* inhibit cramps and diarrhea.
- **For infants, the above OTC preparations are not recommended as the primary treatment. Oral hydration should be tried first (See "Fluids" above).**

- Avoid alcohol, fruits, caffeine drinks, milk and fatty foods.
- Try BRAT: bananas, rice, applesauce and toast.

- Reduce your physical activity; strenuous activity increases bowel activity.

* Because of the risk of Reye's syndrome, aspirin should not be given to or used by children or teenagers who have or are suspected of having flu or chicken pox. Use acetaminophen.

DIZZINESS

Dizziness can have numerous causes. Postural hypotension, a common cause, results from pooling of blood in the legs, causing temporary loss of blood flow to the brain. It can occur after vigorous exercise or when you stand up suddenly. Postural hypotension usually is harmless, unless episodes become more frequent.

Other causes of dizziness and lightheadedness include viral infections such as a cold or influenza. A more intense form of dizziness is vertigo, where a person has difficulty maintaining balance and/or the room seems to "spin." It may be accompanied by vomiting. Vertigo is difficult to diagnose; some cases may be caused by an inner ear infection and should be evaluated by your doctor.

Finally, drug interactions and stress may cause feelings of dizziness. Consult your doctor if you experience dizziness or lightheadedness after taking a new medication. Lightheadedness that comes and goes with stressful episodes generally "comes with the turf" and usually is not a cause for concern. However, you should address the causes of your stress and tension to reduce their frequency or intensity. Refer to p. 15.

CONSULT YOUR DOCTOR IF:

- You experience complete blackouts or loss of consciousness.
- You experience vertigo: balance problems and/or the room seems to spin around.
- You suspect an inner ear infection. Refer to p. 62.
- Lightheadedness or dizziness becomes more intense or frequent over three weeks.
- You're unable to participate in your normal activities because of your lightheadedness.
- You have chest pain or shortness of breath along with the dizziness.

HOMECARE

If physician referral is not recommended at this time, try the following self-care procedures:

- Learn to manage your stress and tension.
- Learn a relaxation technique. Refer to p. 17.
- Avoid "jumping out" of a chair or bed if you have episodes of lightheadedness upon rising.

- After vigorous activity such as running, cool down slowly by walking around for two to three minutes.
- Don't hold your breath when lifting heavy loads. Breathe out when moving the object.

- Carefully follow directions for medication use (OTC and prescription). Be sure not to mix a new medication with other drugs or alcohol without your doctor's permission.

SELF-CARE

57

Fatigue, a lack of energy and a general feeling of being tired, can be linked to such physical causes as a viral infection, lack of sleep and "over-training syndrome" found among many endurance athletes. Fatigue can also be a result of emotional problems such as depression, anxiety or stress. Low blood sugar (hypoglycemia) is rarely a cause for ongoing or chronic fatigue. Most of us have our bouts of tiredness and low energy, lasting a few days. This is usually in reaction to a minor infection, overwork or playing too hard. It is especially important for people with changing work schedules or who "moonlight" to get adequate rest and practice appropriate self-care skills to avoid getting run down.

Recently, a lot of attention has been focused on Chronic Fatigue Syndrome (CFS), a mysterious ailment that leaves its victims with extreme fatigue and flu-like symptoms. Some people have had the illness for more than 10 years, limiting their ability to enjoy a normal life. The cause is unknown and there's no standard treatment.

CONSULT YOUR DOCTOR IF:

• Your fatigue is associated with a cold or flu and HomeCare doesn't reduce symptoms.

• Your fatigue doesn't go away after three weeks.

HOMECARE

If physician referral is not recommended at this time, try the following self-care procedures:

• Get six to eight hours of sleep per night.
• Refer to Insomnia on p. 95.

• Slow down! Modify your schedule if you are "burning the candle at both ends."
• Reduce your workouts for two weeks if you exercise heavily.

• Avoid drinking too much alcohol.
• Reduce your ingestion of caffeine drinks.

• Do not rely on stimulants such as diet pills and amphetamines or illicit drugs such as cocaine to give you "energy."

• Eat balanced meals.
• Drink plenty of fluids, especially during hot, humid days and during strenuous exercise or other work.

• Learn and practice relaxation and stress skills.
• Try to balance your work and play.

SWOLLEN GLANDS

Most cases of swollen glands involve the lymph nodes, or in mumps cases, the salivary glands of the neck.

Lymph nodes are small glands that help your body fight infections such as colds, ear infections and small cuts. They become swollen and hard when an infection occurs and may remain hard after the infection has passed. You can feel lymph nodes in your neck, armpits and groin area. Swollen lymph glands are usually no reason for concern when they are present with minor infections. *Swollen glands (especially in the back of the neck) that are present with fever, sore throat, muscle aches and fatigue may indicate mononucleosis; consult your doctor if these symptoms occur.*

With the mumps, one or both of the salivary glands (located below and forward of the ears) are swollen. Other symptoms include low fever, earache, headache and/or fatigue. Typically a childhood disease, mumps is caused by a virus and cannot be treated directly. Symptom relief, such as controlling fever and getting adequate rest, is the best action to take. Adults should be cautious if they haven't had the mumps: complications such as sterility, although rare, can occur in adult mumps cases.

CONSULT YOUR DOCTOR IF:

- The glands are red, hard and tender to the touch. This usually indicates a bacterial infection.

- The glands do not get smaller after three weeks.

- Swollen glands are accompanied by other symptoms such as fever and weight loss.

- You suspect the mumps: swelling of one or both glands below the ears (classic symptom: person looks like a chipmunk), low fever, fatigue, difficulty swallowing and/or earache.

- You suspect mononucleosis (see symptoms described above).

HOMECARE

If physician referral is not recommended at this time, try the following self-care procedures:

- If lymph nodes are swollen, no treatment is usually required. Watch glands and other symptoms for three weeks.
- Treat other symptoms as they occur, e.g., fever, sore throat, cough. Refer to other conditions discussed in this book.

- Applying warm washcloth can soothe tender lymph nodes.

- If you suspect or have mononucleosis, avoid contact sports since the spleen may be enlarged and could rupture.

SELF-CARE

Colds and influenza (respiratory "flu") are probably the No. 1 reason why people see their doctor. They are also two illnesses that can't be cured by medical treatments; both conditions need to "run their course." Because both are viral infections, they cannot be treated by antibiotics. As the chart below shows, there's little difference between the symptoms of a cold and flu. A person can have all the symptoms of both conditions with either a cold or the flu. Severe symptoms are more likely with flu. The best course of action, except for complications such as pneumonia or ear infections, is to treat the symptoms and reduce the discomfort.

Symptoms:

COLDS	FLU
• Runny nose	• Runny nose
• Sneezing	• Sneezing
• Sore throat, coughing	• Coughing
• Headache	• Headache
• Low-grade fever	• Fever
• Red, itchy eyes	• Fatigue, muscle
• Congested ears	aches

CONSULT YOUR DOCTOR IF:

• You have severe ear pain or trouble breathing or swallowing.

• Cough is severe or lasts more than 10 days.

• Mucus or sputum is thick, smelly, or green or rust-colored.

• Fever stays at 102 degrees F for three days.

* Because of the risk of Reye's syndrome, aspirin should not be given to or used by children or teenagers who have or are suspected of having flu or chicken pox. Use acetaminophen.

60

HOMECARE

If physician referral is not recommended at this time, try the following self-care procedures:

• Drink plenty of fluids such as water, fruit juices and caffeine-free drinks and teas.

• Aspirin, ibuprofen or acetaminophen for fever.*
• Antihistamines or decongestants to help clear nasal congestion.

• Reduce your activity.
• Bed rest may be needed depending on your symptoms.

• Stay warm.
• A vaporizer or humidifier can help keep mucous membranes moist.

• Hot broths such as chicken soup can help clear nasal congestion and soothe the throat.
• Do not neglect trying to eat balanced meals.

• Influenza shots prior to flu season are recommended for adults over age 65 and those under age 65 who suffer from heart and respiratory ailments.
• Wash your hands, especially if a family member has a cold or flu.

ASTHMA

Asthma is an upper respiratory condition caused by a tightening of the muscles of the small breathing tubes (bronchioles) of the lungs. This tightening, called *bronchospasm,* causes labored breathing as the airways become narrowed and restrict air flow. Also, the breathing tubes become inflamed and produce excess mucus which further inhibits breathing. Asthma is more common in children than adults. Research shows however, that many children outgrow this problem once they reach adulthood.

Typical symptoms of an asthma attack include labored breathing (wheezing), shortness of breath, tightness in the chest, and coughing.

Other respiratory ailments, such as allergies (e.g., to pollens, molds, dust, animal dander and certain foods), colds and influenza can trigger asthma attacks. Other factors such as cold air, tobacco smoke, strenuous exercise, air pollution from industrial and auto emissions, pesticides, chemical fumes and stress can cause asthma attacks or make the condition worse.

If you're asthmatic, it's important to be aware of what agents cause your attacks and create ways to avoid or minimize exposure, e.g., staying indoors when the air quality index is above acceptable limits.

Treatment of asthma usually requires an initial medical visit and evaluation. Medication administered through an inhaler may be prescribed to relax bronchospasms during acute attacks or help prevent future attacks.

CONSULT YOUR DOCTOR IF:

- You or your child experience asthma symptoms for the first time.
- Your child has episodes of wheezing.
- You experience an acute asthma attack and HomeCare is not successful in reducing symptoms.
- You cough up sputum that is green, yellow or bloody.

HOMECARE

If physician referral is not recommended at this time, try the following self-care procedures:

- Reduce your activity when an asthma attack occurs.
- Try to remain calm. Stress can increase symptoms.

- Use any prescribed medication only as directed by your doctor.
- Avoid using antihistamines during an asthmatic attack, which may further restrict your airways.

- Drink plenty of clear fluids to help thin and loosen mucus.
- Coffee has been shown to help relieve attacks in some people.

- Stay physically active. Monitor your activity (e.g., exercise intensity) if you have experienced exercise-induced asthma attacks.

- Know what factors (e.g., pollens, smoke, dust, fumes, cold weather, certain foods such as milk and eggs) cause your attacks.
- Avoid these agents or minimize your exposure by keeping your home dust-free.
- If you smoke, try to quit. Avoid smoke-filled areas.
- Try to reduce the stress in your life. Learn a relaxation technique. See p. 17.
- Install an air conditioner in your home and possibly an air filtration system.

Earache is a common problem. It usually occurs in people who have allergies or suffer from a cold.

Earache occurs when the eustachian tube, which equalizes air pressure from the middle ear to the throat, swells shut. When this happens, fluid builds up behind the eardrum, causing pressure and pain. The fluid then can become infected. Indications of ear infections include fever and localized pain. Antibiotics are usually prescribed by your doctor if a bacterial infection is discovered.

Children are especially prone to earache because their eustachian tubes are smaller and swell shut more easily from upper respiratory problems. *Suspect an ear infection if your child has fever and pain and complains of "fullness in the head" and partial hearing loss in the affected ear. In infants, irritability, crying, and rubbing and pulling the ears are possible indications of infection.*

Many earaches occur in the *outer ear*, as in the case of so-called "swimmer's ear" (*the pain is worse when the earlobe is pulled*). Over-the-counter ear drops such as *Auralgan* can be tried at home to treat the infection.

CONSULT YOUR DOCTOR IF:

- You think your infant has an ear infection: rubbing or pulling the ears, crying, irritability and inability to sleep.
- You or an older child experiences ear pain that is severe and lasts for a day.

* Because of the risk of Reye's syndrome, aspirin should not be given to or used by children or teenagers who have or are suspected of having flu or chicken pox. Use acetaminophen.

HOMECARE

If physician referral is not recommended at this time, try the following self-care procedures:

- To help loosen mucus, take a hot shower, use a vaporizer or place a warm washcloth to the ear. Shake head and swallow occasionally.

- In adults: aspirin, ibuprofen or acetaminophen to reduce pain and possible fever. Use as directed.*
- Antihistamines or decongestants may help relieve stuffiness and nasal secretions.
- OTC ear drops such as *Auralgan* can be tried to treat an outer ear infection (e.g., swimmer's ear). Talk to your doctor or pharmacist.

- Drink plenty of water or juices.

- Reduce your activity.

- Ear pain during airplane descent can normally be relieved by holding your nose or blowing your nose while keeping your mouth closed.

Colic is a common problem among infants in their first three months. A colicky baby will cry for long periods, often leading to great stress and many sleepless nights for other family members.

The most common cause of colic is pain in the digestive tract, especially in cases where the crying occurs within a few minutes to a few hours after feeding. Stomach discomfort can result from the baby's swallowing too much air during feeding, an allergy to cow's milk, sugar intolerance or overheated milk.

Stress in the household created by a colicky baby can in turn cause the infant to become more irritable. Trying to keep the household on an even keel may help reduce the worst effects of colic.

You may get some relief for the baby and other family members by trying the suggestions outlined in the HomeCare column. Remember, whatever you do, the problem will probably go away within a few months.

CONSULT YOUR DOCTOR IF:

- Crying is accompanied by diarrhea and/or vomiting. See p. 56.

- You suspect that crying is due to earache. See p. 62.

- The stress in your household becomes overwhelming.

HOMECARE

If physician referral is not recommended at this time, try the following self-care procedures:

- Check to see that baby is being fed enough.
- Stick to the recommended feeding schedule.
- If breastfeeding, decrease the amount of sugar in Mom's diet. Have mother avoid highly spiced foods and alcohol.
- Do not rush feeding.
- Change formula or substitute soy milk for cow's milk if you suspect baby is allergic to cow's milk.

- Check to see that nipple hole on bottle isn't too small. Milk should drip, one drop per second.
- Burp baby after each ounce of milk is taken.

- Don't overheat baby's formula. Keep at body temperature.

SELF-CARE

Dental problems such as tooth decay and gum disease are caused by a buildup of plaque and bacteria around the teeth and gums. The main culprits are infrequent brushing, failure to floss regularly, not using toothpaste that contains fluoride and not seeing your dentist every 6 to 12 months for regular cleaning and inspection. Bacterial buildup creates a film on your teeth called plaque. Plaque attracts sugars that in turn produce acids that can slowly decay the enamel tooth covering. Dental plaque also causes gum disease through the production of acid which inflames the gums or degrades the supporting bone.

Toothache is usually caused by a cavity that has worn through the tooth enamel and has irritated the nerve. A more serious condition is called an abscess. An abscess is a local infection that may include fever, soreness, swelling in the jaw, and redness around the infected tooth. *Your dentist should be notified immediately if you think you have an abscess.*

Bleeding gums are an indication of periodontal disease, which affects the stability of the teeth and jaw. Signs of periodontal disease include reddened, swollen gums; loose teeth; and bleeding on brushing. Though poor oral hygiene is the main cause, pregnancy, medications or diabetes may also increase the risk.

CONSULT YOUR DENTIST IF:

- You have signs of an abscess: soreness, swelling in jaw, redness and fever.
- You have a toothache and you can see or feel a cavity.
- Your gums are bleeding or inflamed, or a tooth is loose.
- Your tooth has been knocked out.

64

HOMECARE

If physician referral is not recommended at this time, try the following self-care procedures:

- To reduce toothache pain, aspirin, ibuprofen, or acetaminophen can be used. Use as directed.*

- Avoid cold beverages when a cavity is present.
- Avoid sugary foods and hard candies.

- Moderate your consumption of foods and beverages that contain sugar.
- Eat green and yellow fruits and vegetables.

- Fluoride treatment or sealants may be recommended by your dentist.
- Visit your dentist every 6 to 12 months for preventive checkups.

- Brush between meals with fluoride toothpaste.
- Floss every day.
- Limit your consumption of sugary foods.

* Because of the risk of Reye's syndrome, aspirin should not be given to or used by children or teenagers who have or are suspected of having flu or chicken pox. Use acetaminophen.

Heartburn

As part of the digestive process, the stomach produces hydrochloric acid. Heartburn is caused when the stomach acid irritates the stomach lining or backs up into the esophagus. Heartburn is a burning sensation just below the breastbone.

Common contributors to heartburn are overeating, alcohol, caffeine, aspirin, ibuprofen, tobacco and emotional stress.

If heartburn is a problem for you, eating smaller portions and more times a day can help reduce it.

Heartburn doesn't usually require medical attention unless it lasts more than three days. Prolonged discomfort may suggest a medical condition such as a hernia or ulcer, which should be evaluated by a doctor.

People having a heart attack may sometimes think they have heartburn. If you experience shortness of breath, or pain in your jaw, radiating down your arm or in your back, seek medical attention immediately. See p. 66.

CONSULT YOUR DOCTOR IF:

- "Heartburn" is combined with shortness of breath, or pain in your jaw, radiating down your arm or in your back.
- Heartburn lasts more than three days.
- You vomit black or bloody material.
- Your stools are black and tar-like.

HOMECARE

If physician referral is not recommended at this time, try the following self-care procedures:

- Avoid vinegar, chocolate, oranges, lemons, grapefruits, pickles and tomatoes.
- Avoid fatty foods and peppermint.
- Avoid alcohol and caffeine.

- Stay mildly active for two hours after eating. An after-dinner walk may aid digestion.

- Wait one to two hours after eating before lying down. If you need to lie down, lie on your left side.
- If you need to rest, keep your shoulders 1 to 2 feet above hips.

- Antacids in liquid or tablet form can relieve gastric discomfort.
- Avoid using aspirin or ibuprofen.

- Avoid tight-fitting clothing and belts that squeeze the abdomen or stomach.

- Avoid overeating.
- Try to manage your levels of stress.
- Don't smoke.

Up to one-third of all heart attacks occur without warning. Therefore, chest pain is a symptom that should never be ignored, especially for people who have a family history of heart disease or have significant risk factors such as high blood pressure, high cholesterol, diabetes, tobacco use, low physical activity and excess body weight.

Chest pain can also be traced to a number of other causes such as heartburn, an ulcer, a hiatus hernia (part of the upper stomach pokes up through the diaphragm), pleurisy (lung infection), blood clots in the lung's blood vessels, acute bronchitis, gallbladder problems, a pulled muscle or a broken rib. A common cause of chest pain is a strained or pulled muscle, usually between the ribs. A sign of this kind of injury: you stick your finger on the site of pain and the pain increases or the site is sensitive to the touch.

The following are classic signs that chest pain may be either a heart attack or angina (an indication that your heart muscle is not getting enough oxygen): *severe pain in the middle of the chest that spreads to the jaw, neck, shoulder, back or arms; shortness of breath; a weak or irregular pulse; sweating; and dizziness.* Not all of these symptoms need to be present with chest pain to indicate a possible heart problem. Therefore, the best practice is to seek medical attention immediately.

SEEK MEDICAL ATTENTION IF:

- You experience one or more of these symptoms: severe pain in the middle of the chest that spreads to the jaw, neck, shoulder, back or arms; shortness of breath; a weak or irregular pulse; sweating or dizziness. **Act immediately.**
- Your chest pain occurs after you have been bedridden due to surgery or some other illness or injury. This may indicate that a blood clot has formed in your lung (It is usually accompanied by shortness of breath).
- Your chest pain is due to a blow to the chest from a fall or other accident, you have difficulty breathing or your ribs are sore to touch.

HOMECARE

If heart attack or another serious condition has been ruled out by your doctor, the following HomeCare treatments can be tried for two common chest pain problems.

- **Heartburn: Refer to p. 65 for a description of Heartburn.**

- **Chest Wall Pain (Pulled Muscle):**

- Avoid activities that require bending, twisting and lifting until pain is reduced.
- Try to breathe with diaphragm only.

- For chest wall pain due to a pulled muscle: aspirin, ibuprofen or acetaminophen may be tried. Rub-on salves such as *Ben-Gay* may also be tried.

- A heating pad over the injured area may help.

STOMACH FLU

Stomach flu (gastroenteritis) is usually a sudden viral infection that brings on stomach cramps, vomiting, nausea and diarrhea. It can also be caused by bacteria found in untreated drinking water (dysentery) or food poisoning (salmonella). The symptoms of gastroenteritis are the body's attempt to cleanse itself of noxious agents such as certain bacteria. Symptoms generally last only one or two days.

Stomach flu can be especially dangerous to infants, small children and the frail elderly because of rapid dehydration caused by vomiting and diarrhea. Excessive vomiting or diarrhea should be carefully watched.

CONSULT YOUR DOCTOR IF:

- Excessive vomiting or diarrhea occurs in infants, small children, the frail elderly or people with other health problems.
- There are signs of dehydration: increased thirst, dark yellow urine, limited urination and skin that may be wrinkled and have no tone.
- Nausea, loss of appetite and general abdominal pain is followed by pain in the lower right part of the abdomen.
- You have a fever of 102 degrees F or higher.
- After only liquids are used, diarrhea continues for more than two days.
- Diarrhea is bloody or black.
- Vomiting continues on and off for more than 12 hours in adults and 4 hours in small children *without* significant improvement.

HOMECARE

If physician referral is not recommended at this time, try the following self-care procedures:

- Choose crushed ice and sips of water for the first few hours.
- Drink clear liquids for the next 24 hours.

- No foods for the first 24 hours.
- Slowly introduce soups and bland foods such as toast and oatmeal on Day 2.

- Aspirin, ibuprofen or acetaminophen for fever. **Do not use aspirin or ibuprofen if you are already vomiting: this will further upset your stomach.***

- Bed rest may be needed.

- Make sure meats are properly stored and prepared.
- Avoid dressings, prepared salads, shellfish (especially raw oysters), poultry and other meats left out more than two hours.

* Because of the risk of Reye's syndrome, aspirin should not be given to or used by children or teenagers who have or are suspected of having flu or chicken pox. Use acetaminophen.

SELF-CARE

Hemorrhoids or "piles" occur when the veins that surround the anus become enlarged and eventually bleed because of increased pressure. Certain conditions increase the risk of hemorrhoids, including being overweight, being constipated, continual straining when trying to defecate, excessive coughing or sneezing, and being pregnant. People in occupations that require long bouts of sitting, such as truck drivers, have a higher incidence of hemorroids.

Typical symptoms of hemorrhoids are rectal pain, itching and bleeding. Rectal bleeding can be a cause for concern, as it may suggest a more serious condition such as an ulcer or cancer. *The blood from hemorrhoids is bright red and may be present on the outside of the stool or on the toilet paper. You should consult your doctor immediately if there's rectal bleeding that makes your stools look black and tar-like. This may be a sign of significant blood loss from higher up in the bowel.*

CONSULT YOUR DOCTOR IF:

- Minor hemorrhoidal bleeding doesn't stop after three weeks of HomeCare.

- Stools are black or tar-like.

- Your child complains of rectal pain or itching, especially at night. This may indicate pinworms.

- Onset of hemorrhoids is associated with a significant change in stool habits for you.

68

HOMECARE

If physician referral is not recommended at this time, try the following self-care procedures:

- Drink plenty of fluids—6 to 8 glasses of water per day.

- Eat more fiber found in fruits, vegetables and whole-grain cereals.

- Use toilet paper gently. Use only white non-perfumed paper that is super soft. Wetting the paper with warm water before use may help as well.

- Of the scores of hemorrhoid medications, none has proved to be more effective than any other. Ask your pharmacist. Consider trying more than one product and see which one gives you the best relief.
- If constipation continues to be a problem despite increasing fliuds and fiber in your diet, consider adding bulk agents containing psyllium (e.g., *Metamucil*) or stool softeners (e.g., *Colace*). Talk to your doctor or pharmacist.

A general misconception about regularity is that daily bowel movements are an indication of well-being. The fact of the matter is that being "regular" is different for each person.

Constipation is defined as difficulty in passing stools, rather than not being able to "go" to the bathroom. Most constipation problems can be fixed by increasing your fluid intake and increasing your consumption of fiber found in fruits, vegetables, cereals and whole-grain breads.

An added benefit of changing your dietary habits is that you will reduce your risk of colon cancer, diverticulosis, polyps and hemorrhoids.

CONSULT YOUR DOCTOR IF:

- Your constipation happens with weight loss, abdominal pain or swelling, or the passage of stools that are pencil-thin or have dark blood, or are black and tar-like.

- Your constipation continues after you have tried HomeCare procedures for more than one week.

HOMECARE

If physician referral is not recommended at this time, try the following self-care procedures:

- Increase your intake of fluids such as water and fruit juices.

- Increase your intake of fruits, whole-grain cereals and breads, and vegetables.

- Increase your physical activity. Brisk walking, aerobic dance and jogging have been shown to increase bowel movements.

- Avoid the frequent use of laxatives. If a laxative is used, try a bulk product that contains fiber. See p. 50, "Over-the-Counter Medications."

- The best way to avoid constipation is to follow dietary recommendations, drink plenty of water and be physically active.
- If constipation continues to be a problem despite increasing fliuds and fiber in your diet, consider adding bulk agents containing psyllium (*e.g.*, *Metamucil*) or stool softeners (e.g., *Colace*). Talk to your doctor or pharmacist

SELF-CARE

Skin abrasions are surface wounds in which layers of the skin are scraped or torn. The primary cause of abrasions is falls; the hands, elbows, knees and hips are the major sites of injury. Team sports such as football, basketball and softball, and activities such as skateboarding, cycling and in-line skating are most frequently associated with abrasion injuries. You should wear gloves and protective knee and elbow pads when engaged in activities for which falls are common. People who work in areas that are slippery (e.g., wet floors, icy walkways) or who climb uneven terrain should be extra careful.

CONSULT YOUR DOCTOR IF:

There are signs of infection:

- Increasing pain or tenderness.

- Swelling and redness.

- Red streaks coming from the injury.

- Presence of pus.

- A fever of 101 degrees F or higher without other causes, such as a cold or flu.

- Date of first tetanus shot is unknown, or wound is not small and clean and your last tetanus shot was more than five years ago.

* Because of the risk of Reye's syndrome, aspirin should not be given to or used by children or teenagers who have or are suspected of having flu or chicken pox. Use acetaminophen.

HOMECARE

If physician referral is not recommended at this time, try the following self-care procedures:

- Rinse the wound with cool water.
- Wash around the wound with soap and water. Avoid getting soap in the wound.
- Use tweezers cleaned in alcohol to remove dirt, glass or gravel that remains in wound.

- If wound covers a large area, oozes blood or is exposed to clothing or dirt, cover with an *occlusive* or *semiocclusive* bandage (see your pharmacist). This dressing keeps the wound moist—reducing scarring and speeding healing.

- Aspirin, ibuprofen or acetaminophen for pain. Use as directed.*

- An ice pack or cool compresses can be tried to help reduce pain.

- Wear protective pads on knees and elbows and gloves when appropriate.
- Beware of slippery or uneven surfaces.
- A tetanus booster shot every 10 years is recommended. See p. 21.

Once a skin cut (laceration) occurs, it's important to determine if the wound requires medical attention because of one of the following conditions: *uncontrolled bleeding; a jagged wound; potential damage to muscles nerves and other soft tissues; possible infection.* Infection usually becomes evident 24 hours after injury. You should also consider seeing your doctor if the cut is too large or deep for you to keep the edges together. Keeping the edges of the wound together helps keep the dirt out and decreases scarring. Stitches provide the best insurance for holding the edges together, but they can cause scarring also. Because of this, your doctor may suggest using butterfly bandages.

You can easily learn to look for signs of infection and the healing process. Ask your doctor. Also, you can learn to remove stitches yourself, which saves both time and money. Ask your doctor for instructions.

CONSULT YOUR DOCTOR IF:

• The wound cannot be closed and bleeding cannot be stopped, the edges won't come together, or the wound is very irregular and there are flaps of tissue.

• Date of first tetanus shot is unknown, or wound is not small and clean and your last tetanus shot was more than five years ago.

• The wound is very dirty or contains foreign material that is not easily washed away.

• There is weakness or numbness below the injury.

• There is a long or deep cut to the face, chest, back, stomach, palm of the hand, or over a joint.

• There are signs of infection:

  - *Increasing pain or tenderness.*

  - *Swelling and redness.*

  - *Red streaks coming away from the injury.*

- *Presence of pus.*

- *A fever of 100 degrees F or higher without another cause, such as cold or flu.*

HOMECARE

If physician referral is not recommended at this time, try the following self-care procedures:

• Rinse the cut with cool water.
• Wash around the wound with soap and water. Avoid getting soap in the wound.
• Use tweezers cleaned in alcohol to remove dirt, glass or gravel that remains in wound.

• Apply pressure directly to wound with clean gauze pad until bleeding has stopped.
• Don't cover unless the cut rubs against clothing or will get dirty.
• If needed, cover with adhesive bandage or larger dressing. Change daily.
• Apply "butterfly" bandage to a deeper cut after bleeding has stopped or slowed.
• Do not pick at the scab.

• Antiseptics such as hydrogen peroxide are not recommended. They can irritate the wound and cause further discomfort.
• Aspirin, ibuprofen or acetaminophen for pain. Use as directed.*

• A tetanus booster shot is recommended every 10 years. See p. 21.

* Because of the risk of Reye's syndrome, aspirin should not be given to or used by children or teenagers who have or are suspected of having flu or chicken pox. Use acetaminophen.

Unlike abrasions and lacerations, which usually are on the skin's surface, puncture wounds can be deep and pose a greater risk of infection. Unfortunately, they're often neglected because of their small size.

Puncture wounds are common to the fingers, hands and the bottom of the feet, and are caused by sharp, pointed objects such as nails, pins, needles, staples and wire. Puncture wounds are common in occupations such as construction, carpentry, medicine (needle sticks) and textile manufacturing.

It is important to thoroughly clean the wound in order to avoid infection, especially with wounds of the hand, head, chest, back or abdomen.

Deep puncture wounds can damage underlying blood vessels, nerves and organs. Indications of additional injury, such as loss of movement, numbness, profuse bleeding (spurting indicates that an artery has been injured) or signs of shock, require immediate medical attention.

CONSULT YOUR DOCTOR IF:

- You cannot stop the bleeding.
- You suspect internal injury to nerves, organs or blood vessels.
- **There are signs of infection:** *increasing pain or tenderness, swelling and redness, red lines coming away from the injury, presence of pus, or a fever of 101 degrees F or higher without another reason, such as cold or flu.*
- Object remains in wound.
- Wound is in hand, head, chest, back or abdomen.
- There are signs of shock: pale, sweating skin, dizziness, rapid/weak pulse.
- It has been more than five years since your last tetanus shot or date of last tetanus shot is not known.

HOMECARE

If physician referral is not recommended at this time, try the following self-care procedures:

- •Rinse the wound with cool water.
- • Wash around the wound with soap and water. Avoid getting soap in the wound.
- • Encourage the wound to bleed, unless serious. Bleeding helps bring material to the surface.

- • To help draw foreign matter and bacteria from wound, soak in warm water 3 times a day for 2 to 4 days.

- • Applying a bandage or sterile dressing is *not* recommended, unless the wound will get dirty or rub against clothing.

- • Aspirin, ibuprofen or acetaminophen for pain. Use as directed.†
- • Antiseptics such as hydrogen peroxide are not recommended. They can irritate the wound and cause further discomfort.

- • A tetanus booster shot every 10 years is recommended. See p. 21.
- • Store sharp objects.
- • Follow procedures when handling syringes and needles.*

* Because of the risk of hepatitis and AIDS through needle sticks, medical personnel should follow infectious disease control measures for the handling of needles and syringes.

†Because of the risk of Reye's syndrome, aspirin should not be given to or used by children or teenagers who have or are suspected of having flu or chicken pox. Use acetaminophen.

Burns are classified in three categories according to their severity:

First-Degree: Limited to the skin's surface, first-degree burns (such as sunburn) are red and painful. They usually do not require medical attention.

Second-Degree: Splitting or blistering of skin is evident, indicating that deeper skin layers have been damaged.

Third-Degree: Severe tissue damage is evident involving the skin, fatty tissue, nerves and other tissues deep below the surface. *Indications of third-degree burns include swelling, skin that is charred or white, and limited pain because nerves have been damaged or destroyed.*

CONSULT YOUR DOCTOR IF:

• Third-degree burns are evident.

• There are extensive second-degree burns or any second-degree burns on the face, hands or feet.

• Pain continues for more than two days.

• There are signs of infection:

- Increasing pain, redness or tenderness.

- Fever of 101 degrees F or greater.

- Area becomes increasingly swollen.

BEWARE OF SUNBURN:

• Exposure to ultraviolet radiation increases your risk of skin cancer. The American Cancer Society urges people to minimize their sun exposure and to use sunscreen with a minimum SPF of 15.

• Examine your skin every three months: look for birthmarks, moles or brown spots that have changed color, size or texture; have an irregular outline; are bigger than a pencil eraser; or continue to itch, scab or bleed. Consult your doctor if you discover any of the above changes. Melanomas and other skin cancers caught early have a high cure rate.

HOMECARE

If physician referral is not recommended at this time, try the following self-care procedures:

• Apply cool compress or cool water to burn area for 5-10 minutes. Continue until pain is reduced.
• **Beware.** Applying ice compress may further damage tissue.

• Aspirin, ibuprofen or acetaminophen to reduce pain Use as directed.*
• *Antibiotic creams have questionable value.*
• Aloe may be tried to help soothe the pain and discomfort.

• Do not cover burn with gauze dressing or bandage, unless area is irritated by clothing or other objects.

• Drink plenty of water.

• Avoid breaking blisters. Do not remove skin.

• Avoid excessive exposure to the sun.
• Use sunblock or SPF 15 suntan lotion.
• Practice fire prevention at work and at home. Assume pots and skillets are hot.

* Because of the risk of Reye's syndrome, aspirin should not be given to or used by children or teenagers who have or are suspected of having flu or chicken pox. Use acetaminophen.

S E L F - C A R E

Millions of Americans go through pollen season suffering from such symptoms as stuffy head; runny nose; watery, itchy eyes; headaches; sneezing; and ticklish throats from post-nasal drip. Allergic rhinitis (hay fever) is the most common respiratory allergy: it is a response to outside substances called *allergens*. Among adults, dust (especially dust mites), animal dander, molds, feathers and pollen are the most common allergens; among infants, food, animal dander and dust are the most common.

For most victims, allergy season is a period of moderate discomfort that you "just grin and sneeze at," hoping that the pollen count stays down. But for others, pollen or dust can cause significant physical problems and be a year-round challenge.

In cases of severe allergy, professional medical consultation is recommended to determine the actual substances that cause the allergic reaction. *Skin or blood tests may be recommended to determine the specific allergen.* People who have severe allergies may go through "hyposensitization" techniques that help them become less sensitive to the allergen through a series of injections.

Most people who have mild to moderate hay fever can follow the HomeCare procedures listed. Whenever possible, avoiding the known allergens is the best course of action.

CONSULT YOUR DOCTOR IF:

- You have difficulty breathing or severe wheezing.
- Nasal discharge is green or yellow.
- Your life has become miserable due to the symptoms.
- The symptoms have become much worse.

HOMECARE

If physician referral is not recommended at this time, try the following self-care procedures:

- Antihistamines to help relieve symptoms. *Use with caution; read labels.*
- Nasal decongestants for stuffy head.
- Cough drops for post-nasal drip.

- Use tissue or handkerchief to gently blow mucus from nose. Do not blow hard: ear infection or bloody nose could result.

- Cover nose and mouth with mask when doing household chores that have worsened symptoms in the past, such as cutting the lawn and dusting.

- Keep room air moist through the use of a humidifier, especially in bedrooms.
- If you're allergic to molds, consider using an air conditioner with an electostatic filter during the summer.

- You may need more rest when allergy strikes.

- If possible, avoid contact with allergens such as flowers, grasses, specific foods and dust.
- Keep house pets out of bedrooms. Try to keep your pet clean and groomed.

FOOD ALLERGY

Symptoms of a food allergy include fainting, *swelling of the lips and mouth; hives; itching on the palms and soles of the feet or other parts of the body; wheezing; runny nose; and gastrointestinal distress such as cramping, vomiting or diarrhea.* Food allergies can affect all age groups but are most frequent among children.

As with any allergy, avoiding contact with the allergen is the best self-care procedure. If you suspect you have a food allergy, it is important to try to identify the food agent. For example, if biting into an apple causes your throat to swell slightly, you may be allergic to either the apple or something sprayed on the apple. You may find that eating a slice without the skin produces no symptoms: you have narrowed down the cause further. Special food preparation (e.g., peeling the apple) can help you avoid a reaction.

Food allergies in children have been linked to a number of foods such as peanuts (the worst), strawberries, citrus fruit, seafood, wheat, eggs, nuts, beef and especially cow's milk. There is some evidence that suggests that breastfeeding helps protect infants from future allergies, and that early exposure to cow's milk may increase the chances of asthma later in life.

CONSULT YOUR DOCTOR IF:

- You have an allergic reaction that produces severe breathing problems, wheezing or fainting.
- Other symptoms listed above are severe.

HOMECARE

If physician referral is not recommended at this time, try the following self-care procedures:

- Antihistamines may be used for mild to moderate reactions.
- Treat symptoms as indicated in other sections.

- Use tissue or handkerchief to gently blow mucus from nose. Do not blow hard: ear infection or bloody nose could result.

- Reduce your activity when an allergic reaction happens.

- You may need to rest after an allergic reaction.

- Soybean milk substitute may be tried if infant shows intolerance to cow's milk.
- Avoid foods that may cause a reaction: track down possible offenders.

- Breastfeeding may build resistance to some allergies in infants.
- If known, avoid foods that may cause allergic reactions.
- Avoid foods more likely to cause allergies when starting infants on solids.

SELF-CARE

Contact dermatitis is an allergic skin rash caused by an external chemical agent that comes in contact with the skin. Common sources of dermatitis are poison ivy, poison oak and poison sumac; insecticides; solvents; caustic industrial chemicals; cosmetics; jewelry; and synthetic fibers. *Dermatitis often is characterized by the outline of the offending agent, such as the elastic bands from undergarments, or is localized on one part of the body.* If a localized rash appears, it's important to identify the possible cause:

- Have you been close to poison ivy, poison sumac or poison oak?
- Have you changed laundry detergents, soaps, deodorants, shampoos or cosmetics?
- Have you been exposed to insecticides or other chemicals?
- Have you purchased new clothing or jewelry?

CONSULT YOUR DOCTOR IF:

- The rash does not improve after one week.
- The rash becomes bright red, seeps pus or has red streaks that come away from the infected area.
- You become feverish.
- Itching is severe and does not respond to HomeCare procedures.
- Rash is near your eyes, especially if the eyes are reddened.

76

HOMECARE

If physician referral is not recommended at this time, try the following self-care procedures:

- Use soap and water to remove chemicals or other agents. A non-lipid cleaning solution such as *Cetaphil* is better than soap. For oily substances, use rubbing alcohol, then use soap and water.
- Follow guidelines for exposure to chemicals or insecticides.

- Apply cool compresses of Burrow's solution for cases of poison ivy, oak or sumac. Burrow's solution can be purchased at your local pharmacy as an OTC. Use as directed.
- Antihistamines to reduce itching. Use as directed.

- If practical, do not cover. Expose rash to air. Don't scratch it for relief. Scratching can spread the rash and cause infection.

- Use cosmetics that are hypo-allergenic.

- Avoid areas that are infested with poison ivy, sumac or oak.
- Handle chemicals with care.

People react differently to insect bites or stings. Most experience a localized allergic reaction that is limited to the bite area. Common symptoms of a localized reaction are swelling, itching and redness. *A generalized (systemic) reaction is serious and life threatening. Symptoms include wheezing, tightness in the throat, shortness of breath, hives covering the body, swollen eyes and possible abdominal pain.*

Individuals who work or play outdoors and have had a generalized reaction should be equipped with a kit that contains epinephrine. *It is also wise to alert your family, friends and coworkers to your problem, the related symptoms and the use of your epinephrine kit in the event that you are incapacitated.* It is important to seek medical emergency assistance as soon as possible.

Another cause of concern is the threat of **Lyme disease** spread by the deer tick (Ixodes). Proper coverage (tick repellent and clothing) and avoidance of grassy and wooded areas is the best defense. Doctor referral is recommended if you suspect a tick bite and you experience any of the following symptoms: *a bull's-eye rash, flu-like symptoms (muscle aches, fever and fatigue), swelling of the joints (especially the knees), shortness of breath, temporary facial paralysis, heart irregularities, and/or memory and concentration problems.*

CONSULT YOUR DOCTOR IF:

- You suffer a generalized reaction as described above.
- A localized reaction does not improve within 72 hours.
- There are signs of infection after a localized reaction subsides (usually after 24 hours: fever, redness and swelling and the presence of pus).
- You suspect you may have Lyme disease (see the symptoms listed above).

HOMECARE

If physician referral is not recommended at this time, try the following self-care procedures:

- Apply ice or cold packs immediately following bite or sting.

- Reduce your activity immediately if you begin experiencing a generalized reaction.

- To relieve itching, an antihistamine can be used as directed. Don't scratch the area to relieve itching. This can cause infection.

- Carry a kit containing epinephrine if you suffer generalized reactions and you regularly work or play outdoors. Instruct family and coworkers on its use, in case you're incapicitated. Talk to your doctor.

- Avoid places where insect bites and stings are more likely to happen.
- Use insect repellents that contain diethyltoluamide (DEET).
- Avoid brightly colored clothes, as they may attract bees.
- To help prevent Lyme disease, avoid high grass and wooded areas. Avoid wearing shorts or skirts. Inspect your pets before allowing them in the house. Remove a tisk with tweezers or tissue. Grab the mouth parts; don't squeeze the body. Disinfect bite with alcohol. Wash your hands with soap and water.

SELF-CARE

77

SELF-CARE

Injury to the eyes is a major risk in certain jobs such as manufacturing, carpentry, yard maintenance and mining. Work around the house and recreational activities can increase the risk of dirt and other small objects getting into the eye. The use of shatterproof glasses or goggles is your first line of defense.

When the eye is affected by a foreign object, it's wise to take the problem seriously. First, try to locate the object in the eye. If the object is located in the corner or close to the lower lid, moisten the twisted tip of a tissue and gently dab the object. This should lift the object from the eye.

Gently wash the eye out with water, saline solution used for contact lenses, or a commercial eye wash solution. Using your thumb and forefinger, carefully and gently grasp the eyelid above the eyelash and repeatedly lift it away from the eye. This allows the natural fluids to wash the eye or help move an object toward the edges.

You should never rub the eye. This may cause the cornea to be scratched and increase the chances of infection. If you have difficulty in locating the object or removing the object, see your doctor immediately.

CONSULT YOUR DOCTOR IF:

- Your eye is bloody or torn.
- The object appears to be stuck in the eye.
- HomeCare procedures have failed to remove the object.
- You have vision problems or pain and discomfort 24 hours after removing the object.

HOMECARE

If physician referral is not recommended at this time, try the following self-care procedures:

- Use a moistened, twisted tip of a tissue to remove object in the corner of the eye or close to lower lid. Gently dab and lift object from eye.

- Gently wash the eye with water, contact lens solution or a commercial eye wash solution. Repeat lifting eyelid from eye to promote eye fluids. Keep eye wash in your medicine cabinet.

- In cases where there is still *minor* discomfort after the object has been removed and eye cleaned, cover the eye with a gauze patch for 24 hours.

- Wear shatterproof safety glasses or goggles in jobs or tasks that expose you to dirt, wood splinters/sawdust or metal particles.

CHEMICALS IN THE EYE

Exposure of the eyes to chemicals is a serious risk among employees who work with solvents and other substances. Home products such as cleaning products, paints and fertilizers pose their own risks to both adults and children. *Immediate action is required when a chemical agent is accidentally splashed into the eye.*

The best way to prevent exposure is to wear proper eye protection (shatterproof glasses or goggles) and to follow procedures in handling caustic agents.

CONSULT YOUR DOCTOR IF:

• You have been exposed to a strong chemical agent such as an acid (e.g., sulfuric acid) or a corroding agent (e.g., lye). *Flush the eye with water immediately and continue for at least 15 minutes. Go to the nearest treatment center.*

• You experience symptoms such as continued burning or irritation in the eye, blurred or poor vision, extreme redness or whiteness, watering or discharge.

• HomeCare procedures fail to give relief and eye continues to hurt after 30 minutes of treatment.

HOMECARE

If physician referral is not recommended at this time, try the following self-care procedures:

• Flush eye immediately with water. Don't flush with head back. Keep head down: either immerse in sink or splash water up into eye. Flush under lids.

• Wear glasses or goggles.
• For chemicals, follow safety guidelines as specified by manufacturer. Read labels.

SELF-CARE

Arthritis is a painful condition of the joints. *Common symptoms include inflammation, heat and redness in the affected area, and stiffness and difficulty in moving the joint(s) through the full range of motion.* There are more than 100 kinds of arthritis. However, most arthritis cases fall within four general categories:

• Osteoarthritis. A degeneration of the smooth cartilage that forms the surface of a joint, e.g., knee or shoulder. Osteoarthritis is the most common form of arthritis. It can result from an injury to the joint, or from repeated force placing an unnatural load on the joint. Important note: *There is no evidence that moderate exercise such as walking, jogging and cycling increases the risk of arthritis if the activity is practiced with proper technique and equipment.*

• Rheumatoid Arthritis. Inflammation and deterioration of the joint membrane (usually in the fingers and toes). Rheumatoid arthritis is called an autoimmune condition, because the body's immune system destroys its own tissue. Other body organs such as the heart, kidneys, lungs, skin and eyes can be damaged.

• Gout. Acute, severe pain and swelling in one joint (e.g., big toe) that is caused by a buildup of uric acid crystals in the fluid that bathes the joint.

• Ankylosing Spondylitis. A degeneration of the joints that support and are part of the spinal column.

CONSULT YOUR DOCTOR IF:

• You experience inflamed joint(s) with fever.

• You experience joint pain with flu-like symptoms (especially if you suspect a tick bite).

• Pain prevents you from moving the joint through its range of motion without extreme discomfort.

• You have a new, sudden onset of pain and swelling in a joint.

HOMECARE

If physician referral is not recommended at this time, try the following self-care procedures:

• Rest affected area when you experience flare-ups of inflammation.

• Apply heating pads or hot towels over affected area for 20 minutes.

• Aspirin or ibuprofen to reduce pain and inflammation. **Do not use aspirin**, if flu-like symptoms are present in chidren or teenagers.

Try to gently move stiff joints through their range of motion, three times a day/10 to 20 times per set.
• Water exercises and swimming are excellent activities for many arthritic conditions. Consult your doctor before trying if you're currently under treatment.

• Try to keep body weight within recommended range. Excess body weight can place added stress on already weak joints.
• If affected person has difficulty with everyday activities (e.g., opening doors, opening jars, holding utensils) consider purchasing user-friendly home aides to assist.

• Try to avoid heavy, repetitive strain on joints.
• Use the proper equipment and techniques in work and play. Practice proper work posture.
• Avoid tick-infested areas that may expose you to Lyme disease. See p. 77.

Broken Bones

Broken bones are classified in two categories: 1) simple fractures, where the broken bone does not penetrate the skin; and 2) compound fractures, where the bone is forced through the skin, with external injury and bleeding present.

You should consult your doctor if you suspect a bone fracture. However, every suspected fracture does not require immediate medical attention. Medical attention for simple fractures such as those to the fingers can be delayed for 24 hours if the affected area is immobilized with a splint or by taping the injured finger to the healthy finger next to it. Swelling can be treated with ice packs; pain can be reduced with aspirin or ibuprofen.

Immediate medical care should be taken for shock, which is a serious and life threatening reaction to injury. Signs of shock include skin that is cold, pale and clammy; rapid/weak pulse rate; increased thirst and dizziness; or fainting. Follow these first-aid procedures:

Lay the victim flat, elevate feet 4 inches from ground (unless injury is to head or chest). If bleeding is present, slow or stop bleeding through direct pressure to wound. Call 911 or seek medical assistance.

CONSULT YOUR DOCTOR IMMEDIATELY IF:

- A compound fracture is evident: the bone is sticking through the skin.

- There are signs of shock. See above.

- The injury is deformed, sensitive to the touch, painful to move, shows acute swelling, is discolored or cold, or has no feeling.

- The injury is to the neck or back, with the victim unable to move.

HOMECARE

If physician referral is not recommended at this time, try the following self-care procedures:

- If fracture is questionable and no serious medical conditions are present, rest and immobilize area for 24 to 48 hours. See doctor if condition doesn't improve.

- Ice packs can be used in first 24 to 48 hours if fracture is questionable.

- Aspirin or ibuprofen to reduce pain and inflammation.

Your weekend softball game ends suddenly when, rounding first base, you feel acute pain in the back of your thigh. Or you're playing catch with the kids when you suddenly feel a tear in your shoulder. These injuries are examples of muscle strains, often called muscle pulls.

Strains are tears or stretches in the muscle fibers or the tendons that connect muscles to bones. *Common symptoms include pain, spasm, point tenderness and weakness in the injured area.* Strains can range from relatively mild injuries, with some muscle fibers being torn, to large muscle tears with swelling and hemorrhage (internal bleeding) present.

Causes of muscle strain include:

• muscular imbalance, where one side of the joint is stronger than the other, or the opposite muscle doesn't relax while the other contracts. This can be traced in most cases to either a lack of conditioning or overtraining one muscle group vs. an opposing muscle group, e.g., front of the thigh (quadriceps) vs. the back of the thighs (hamstrings).

• muscle fatigue, which places additional stress on the muscle and connective tissue.

The more active you are, the greater your risk of injury. Poorly conditioned people also are at risk when they suddenly engage in strenuous activity without proper pre-conditioning.

It's therefore important for the "weekend warrior" and the serious marathoner alike to take the time to adequately prepare for an activity. Listen to your body. If something hurts, your body is telling you something is not right. Ease up or stop.

Remember. Properly warm up and cool down, and ease into your activity. Take the time to get in shape before you plunge in your activity.

CONSULT YOUR DOCTOR IF:

• There's excessive swelling, bruising and/or tenderness in the injured area.

• Pain prevents you from moving.

HOMECARE

If physician referral is not recommended at this time, try the following self-care procedures:

• Reduce your activity. Avoid movements that place stress on injured area.

• Apply cold pack or ice massage 20 minutes on, 20 minutes off for two hours. Continue for 24 to 48 hours after injury.
• Heating pads, whirlpools or analgesic balms may be tried on third day if swelling is gone.

• Apply elastic bandage to injured area.

• Elevate injured area for 24 to 48 hours depending on severity of injury.

• Aspirin or ibuprofen to reduce pain and inflammation. Use as directed.

• Try slow, gentle stretches if injury is a mild strain. Avoid stretching for a few days if injury is moderate or severe. However, do general movements (e.g., slow walking, gentle arm circles) that promote circulation to the injured area.
• Properly condition for your activity, including properly warming up and cooling down.
• Use weight training to achieve adequate levels of strength in major muscle groups.

NECK PAIN

The most common reason for neck pain is poor posture at work or at home. At work, sitting for prolonged periods of time in a fixed position can lead to occasional stiffness or cramping. This is especially common among people who do word processing or data entry. At home, a poor sleeping position is a major culprit. Sleeping on a firmer mattress or changing to a thinner pillow will usually correct the problem.

Many people respond to emotional stress by tensing the neck muscles. Over time this can lead to both neck pain and headaches.

Neck pain can also be caused by blows to the head and neck, as in the case of falls and motor vehicle accidents. Sudden twisting or snapping of the head can lead to muscle strain and ligament damage. A pinched nerve can also be a consequence of neck injury or arthritis.

A serious, life-threatening situation that demands immediate medical attention is the suspicion of meningitis. Symptoms of meningitis include fever, headache and a stiff neck that prevents a person from touching the chin to the chest.

In most cases of occasional neck pain, self-care, modifying your work posture and taking periodic rest breaks usually correct the problem and prevents reoccurrences.

CONSULT YOUR DOCTOR IF:

- Neck pain is related to an acute injury or blow to the head.

- You have a fever, headache and a stiff neck that prevents you from touching your chin to your chest.

- Pain radiates down one arm or you experience tingling in your hands.

- Pain does not lessen after seven days.

HOMECARE

If physician referral is not recommended at this time, try the following self-care procedures:

- Sleep on a firm mattress.
- If you have pain in the morning, use a thinner pillow or none at all.
- Make sure your work posture is correct.

- Aspirin or ibuprofen to relieve pain and inflammation. Use as directed. Avoid using aspirin in children and teenagers if neck pain is related to flu or chicken pox.

- Try hot showers, hot compresses or a heating pad.

- Take a bath towel, fold lengthwise to form a 4-inch band. Wrap around neck before bedtime.

- Stay physically active.
- Gently drop your head to your chest and from one side to the other. Do not tip head back.

- Practice proper posture when doing repeated work tasks such as word processing and lifting. Take rest breaks every hour.
- Learn a general relaxation technique. See p. 15.
- Massage your neck muscles.

Elbow pain can be traced to a number of causes: (1) bursitis, an inflammation of the fluid-filled bursa sac at the tip of the elbow; (2) "tennis elbow," an irritation of the tendon that slides over the elbow joint; (3) pain from a fall in which the arm is hyper-extended (e.g., sticking the arm out to break a fall); or (4) direct trauma, such as chipping a bone or tearing the soft tissues around the joint.

In most cases, elbow pain results from repetitive movements that place strain on tendons, the bursa and soft tissues that support the elbow. Tennis elbow usually is caused by repeated twisting or rolling of the forearm, wrist and hands. Tennis elbow is common in sports such as tennis or baseball (pitching), and in jobs that require twisting movements such as assembly and carpentry (e.g., using a screwdriver) or meat packing (e.g., cutting).

When pain is linked to repetitive motion, it's important to:

- use equipment that fits properly (e.g., a screwdriver handle that fits the hand or a tennis racquet with a grip and weight appropriate for you).

- keep your forearm muscles strong.

- take regular stretch breaks, especially if you do repetitive tasks.

- use the proper technique in performing the task that requires repetitive movements.

CONSULT YOUR DOCTOR IF:

• You suspect a fracture or dislocation of elbow due to fall or direct injury.

• You cannot move your elbow (elbow seems locked).

• There are signs of infection: *fever, redness, heat and swelling in elbow.*

• There is numbness or weakness in the hand.

• Pain is not reduced after two weeks of HomeCare.

HOMECARE

If physician referral is not recommended at this time, try the following self-care procedures:

• Aspirin or ibuprofen may help reduce inflammation and discomfort. Use as directed.

• For first 48 hours, apply ice packs to elbow for 20 minutes at a time.
• Heating pads are not recommended.

• Rest the elbow for one to two days; a sling may help.
• Avoid repetitive movements and stress on elbow joint.

• After 48 hours, move elbow through full range of movement every hour.
• Avoid or reduce painful activity.
• Strengthen and stretch forearm and shoulder muscles.

• Use proper tools and equipment.
• Use proper posture and technique when doing repetitive tasks.
• Strengthen and stretch forearm and shoulder muscles.

WRIST PAIN

The wrist consists of eight bones forming a stable platform that allows the hand to move freely. When the hand is bent back or dropped down, it places stress on the tendons and nerves that pass through the wrist. If the wrist is locked in either position for extended periods, damage and pain can occur. Therefore, the best hand position for word processing or data entry keeps the hands in a flat position.

A serious wrist condition called Carpal Tunnel Syndrome (CTS) has become one of the fastest growing occupational injuries. CTS commonly occurs among people whose work requires them to do repetitive movements with their hands. *Symptoms of CTS include pain in wrist and forearm; weakness and loss of mobility in the hand; numbness in the fingers, except the little and ring fingers; and tingling in the fingers when the wrist is tapped.*

Other causes of wrist pain include rheumatoid arthritis, osteoporosis and injuries due to falls or trauma.

CONSULT YOUR DOCTOR IF:

- You have fever, swelling or severe pain even at rest.
- There is weakness, numbness or tingling in your fingers that doesn't go away after 48 hours of following HomeCare suggestions.
- Your wrist is deformed, discolored or sore to the touch after an accident.

HOMECARE

If physician referral is not recommended at this time, try the following self-care procedures:

- Chronic wrist pain requires rest from the activity that caused the problem; one to two weeks is usually adequate.

- Aspirin or ibuprofen may help inflammation. Use as directed.

- A splint from a drugstore or medical supply house could be tried for a few days and then used at night for three weeks.

- Strengthen forearm muscles. Squeeze tennis ball 20 times, three times per day.
- Stretch fingers and wrists every hour. ***Do not do these exercises if you experience pain in your wrists or hands.***
- Use appropriate posture and technique during repetitive tasks.

Back pain is very common. It's estimated that 70 to 80 percent of all adults have had at least one episode of back pain. The good news is that the majority of all back pain episodes will go away within a few days, regardless of the treatment. However, back pain is still a major problem. For some people, pain management is an ongoing concern.

Most lower back pain is due to the spasm of the muscles that support the spinal column. Very few back problems are due to a "slipped disc," where the disc bulges out and irritates the nerve roots.

Back problems can be traced to poor posture, poor lifting techniques, repetitive twisting movements, sitting for extended periods, vibration from vehicles and machinery, poor physical conditioning and stress. Refer to p. 114 for more information on back care.

CONSULT YOUR DOCTOR IF:

- Injury is due to a fall or being hit in the back and prevents the victim from moving legs. Keep person still and call for emergency care.

- Pain or numbness moves into the leg or foot.

- Pain is *severe* even though you can still move.

- Low back pain happens with other physical symptoms such as painful or frequent urination, menstrual pain, flu, gastrointestinal distress or abdominal pain.

- Low back pain is associated with loss of control of bladder or bowels.

- HomeCare procedures fail to provide relief after 72 hours.

- Low back pain is associated with weakness of any muscles in the leg or foot.

H O M E C A R E

If physician referral is not recommended at this time, try the following self-care procedures:

- Limit your activity.
- For severe back pain, rest on a firm mattress or the floor with your back flat for first 24 to 48 hours. A pillow under the knees also may provide relief.

- *If you experience an acute injury*, apply ice packs for 20 minutes every hour, for first 24 to 48 hours. Beware of numbness and white skin (frostbite).
- Heating pads are not recommended for first 48 hours for acute injuries. Heat can be used for mild pain and discomfort.

- Aspirin or ibuprofen to reduce pain and inflammation. Use as directed.

- Practice proper lifting techniques. See p. 115.
- Keep back, leg and abdominal muscles conditioned. See p. 116.
- Use proper work posture.

The primary function of the knee is to support weight and movement in a forward direction. Actions that twist or put excessive force on the inside or outside of the knee joint can easily stretch or tear the ligaments and wear away or tear cartilage that support and protect the knee. In many cases, surgery is done as a last resort.

Knee pain can be caused by a repeated force placed on the knee, such as during prolonged kneeling. Over time, the bursae (protective fluid sacs) of the knee can become inflamed and cause pain. Knee pads are recommended for jobs that require kneeling.

Another cause of knee pain is so-called "runner's knee," which is a gradual wearing of the cartilage behind the kneecap. Runner's knee is usually traced to weak thigh muscles, running on crowned roads (roads that slope from middle to edge) and an excessive inside rolling of the foot (pronation) when it makes contact with the ground. Strength training, changing to a flat running surface and anti-pronation running shoes or special inserts (orthotics) help prevent the problem.

CONSULT YOUR DOCTOR IF:

- You have an injury that prevents you from walking or putting full weight on the injured leg, or your knee cannot be straightened or wobbles from side to side.

- Your knee has rapid, extensive swelling, with or without injury.

- Knee pain is accompanied by fever.

- You have dull pain or discomfort related to jogging, cycling or prolonged kneeling, that's behind or around the kneecap and doesn't go away after four weeks of HomeCare.

- You have pain or swelling in your calf muscle, below the back of your knee.

HOMECARE

If physician referral is not recommended at this time, try the following self-care procedures:

- Avoid taking part in activities that may place stress on the knee.
- To prevent your knee from "locking," don't sleep with pillow under knee.
- A cane or crutches may help to take weight off the injured knee.

- Aspirin or ibuprofen may help to reduce pain and inflammation. Use as directed.

- Ice pack for first 24 to 48 hours after injury: 20 minutes on, 20 minutes off.
- Hot bath or whirlpool may help thereafter.

- Avoid keeping knee in a fixed position for extended periods of time. Every hour, gently straighten and flex the injured leg.
- Once healed, strengthen the front and back thigh muscles. Consult a sports trainer. Walking or pool exercises are excellent options.

- Wear knee pads if your job requires prolonged kneeling.
- If you jog or run, wear the proper shoes; avoid uneven surfaces.

SELF-CARE

The ankle is a hinge joint that connects the lower leg bones with the foot through many tough fiber cords called ligaments. Because of these ligament "bridges," the ankle is quite strong and able to handle a lot of force and movement.

If you twist your ankle, it often can result in an injury to these ligaments. *An ankle strain occurs when the ligaments are stretched beyond their normal limit. An ankle sprain occurs when the ligaments are partially or completely torn.*

You can twist your ankle by stopping suddenly or just putting your foot down the wrong way (e.g., turning it in). People in occupations such as construction, ground maintenance and surveying are prone to twisted ankles, as are "weekend warriors" who engage in softball, basketball and racquet sports.

If you've had a severe ankle injury, your first concern is to determine if a fracture has occurred. Indications of a possible fracture include: swelling, discoloration (black and blue), and a joint that is deformed or bent in an odd way. If a fracture is suspected, keep the ankle immobilized, apply ice to the injured area and seek medical attention immediately.

Most ankle injuries are not fractures or severe sprains, and can be treated using the self-care procedures listed under HomeCare.

CONSULT YOUR DOCTOR IF:

- You suspect a fracture. See above.
- Pain prevents you from placing weight on the ankle 24 hours after the injury occurred.
- You are unable to bear weight on the ankle or pain continues after 72 hours.

HOMECARE

If physician referral is not recommended at this time, try the following self-care procedures:

Rest ankle for 12 to 24 hours; avoid putting weight on it.
- Keep ankle elevated if swelling occurs.
- Expect limited range of motion for two weeks or longer.

- Aspirin or ibuprofen can be used to reduce pain and inflammation. Use as directed.

- Apply ice pack to ankle to minimize swelling, ice area for 20 minutes, rest for 20 minutes. Continue for two to three hours or when swelling is reduced.

- Wrap ankle firmly in elastic bandage if injury has significant swelling. Do not wrap too tight. It should provide comfort, not increase the pain. Keep on for 24 to 48 hours.

- Once pain and swelling have subsided, slowly rotate, flex and extend ankle three times/day to prevent adhesions.

- Learn strengthing exercises if you have a history of weak ankles. Consult a physical therapist or athletic trainer for advice.
- Wear shoes or work boots that fit you and your activity. Look for firm ankle support before purchasing footwear.

MENSTRUAL CRAMPS

Cramping in the lower abdomen is a common problem during a women's menstrual period. *Other symptoms such as headache, backache, thigh pain, diarrhea, constipation, dizziness and nausea are also common.*

Menstrual cramps are caused by natural substances called prostaglandins that are found in higher concentrations during the menstrual period, and can lead to severe cramping for some women. In many cases, cramping can be reduced through HomeCare.

CONSULT YOUR DOCTOR IF:

- Cramping does not stop when your period is over.
- You have a fever, diarrhea or a rash during your period.
- Menstrual bleeding has been unusually heavy for several months.
- After experiencing "normal periods," you suddenly have painful cramping.
- Cramping occurs with signs of major intestinal problems such as black, tarry stools, or blood in the stools themselves.

PREVENTING TOXIC SHOCK SYNDROME

Toxic Shock Syndrome (TSS) is a potentially fatal bacterial infection that is linked with superabsorbent tampons and contraceptive sponges and diaphragms.

Symptoms of TSS include a sudden high fever, headache, vomiting, diarrhea, weakness and redness of the skin, mouth and vagina. Immediate medical attention is required.

HOMECARE

If physician referral is not recommended at this time, try the following self-care procedures:

- Ibuprofen is a very effective treatment for menstrual cramps. Aspirin can also be used. Use as directed.

- Take a hot bath; try to relax.
- Apply heating pads or hot water bottles to relax muscles and reduce cramping.

- Reduce your intake of salt and sodium products, especially the week prior to starting your period.

- Physical activity has been shown to help reduce cramping for some women.

- To help relax, try herbal teas (e.g., chamomile).
- Avoid caffeinated foods (e.g., chocolate) and drinks, which may increase tension and irritability.

- Try sanitary napkins instead of tampons. Change them often.
- Regular physical activity may help reduce cramping episodes.
- To help prevent TSS, avoid using superabsorbent tampons, especially if you have light periods. Use tampons with the lowest absorbency. Change every four to six hours.
- Do not keep contraceptive sponges or diaphragms in longer than 24 hours. Use as directed.

PREMENSTRUAL SYNDROME (PMS)

Premenstrual syndrome (PMS), which is the result of hormonal changes in the body prior to menstruation, is an unwelcome part of the menstrual cycle for many women. PMS can be mild for some, severe for others. *Physical symptoms associated with PMS include weight gain, headaches, acne, bloating, breast tenderness, diarrhea or constipation, dizziness and fatigue.*

Emotional symptoms include mood swings, increased tension and anger, irritability, sadness and unexplained crying. These physical and emotional changes usually take place seven to 10 days prior to menstruation and may disappear just before or at the start of menstruation.

CONSULT YOUR DOCTOR IF:

• Your symptoms are severe for several months and do not improve with the HomeCare guidelines listed below.

HOMECARE

If physician referral is not recommended at this time, try the following self-care procedures:

• Decrease sugar and sodium intake, increase your protein intake.
• Talk to your doctor about taking a vitamin B6 (pyridoxine) supplement and extra magnesium.

• For menstrual cramps try ibuprofen. Aspirin may also be used, but ibuprofen is usually more effective. Use as directed.

• Discuss your PMS problems with your partner. Try to work together to deal with emotional and physical changes.
• To reduce ankle swelling, keep legs elevated.

• Limit your intake of caffeine found in coffee, tea, chocolate and cola drinks. Caffeine can increase irritability and breast tenderness.
• Avoid alcohol, especially if depression is one of your symptoms.

• Try to get extra sleep a few days before you usually experience symptoms.
• Learn a relaxation technique to use when feeling tense. See p. 17.
• Soak in a warm bath tub to help relax aching muscles.

• Exercise three to five days a week with such activities as brisk walking, cycling or swimming.

Vaginitis

Vaginitis (inflammation of the vagina) usually results in one or more of the following symptoms: *abnormal discharge, itching and pain (especially during intercourse). Infection is the most common cause of vaginitis.*

When the vagina is irritated due to an infection, friction caused by intercourse usually makes the condition worse. *Therefore, intercourse is not recommended until the infection has been treated.* Vaginal dryness also can cause pain and irritation during intercourse. A lubricant such as *K-Y Jelly or Replens* can help reduce vaginal dryness.

Infections of the vagina can be caused by yeast (also called monilia or candida), trichomonas, chlamydia, gonorrhea and herpes. Although yeast infections are rarely spread during sex, the other four infections are sexually transmitted.

Yeast infections usually cause itching and a discharge that is not foul smelling (it may smell like baking bread) and looks a bit like cottage cheese. You are at a greater risk for yeast infections if you have diabetes, use birth control pills, are on hormone replacement therapy or are taking antibiotics. Medications (which have a very good cure rate), are now available over the counter for treating yeast infections.

CONSULT YOUR DOCTOR IF:

- The problem is vaginal dryness, and friction, vaginal symptoms and discomfort don't go away after one month of stopping tampon use and using lubrication (e.g. *K-Y Jelly*).

- You or your sexual partner have symptoms that suggest a sexually transmitted disease, e.g., painful discharge, pain on urination.

- It's the first vaginal infection you have ever had.

- You have tried over-the-counter medication for one episode of a possible yeast infection with no success.

HOMECARE

If physician referral is not recommended at this time, try the following self-care procedures:

- Reduce your intake of sugar. If you have diabetes, be sure to watch your blood sugar levels.

- Consider using an over-the-counter vaginal medication (e.g., *Monistat*) for one episode if you have typical symptoms of a yeast infection (monilia vaginitis): itching, a cheesy discharge that may smell like baking bread, no pain and no fever. Use as directed and see your doctor if symptoms persist.

- Use tampons only during times of heavy menstrual flow, if at all. See p. 89.
- For vaginal dryness and friction, use a lubricant during sexual intercourse. Do not use petroleum jelly with condoms; use a water-based lubricant such as *K-Y Jelly* instead.
- Use only water when washing around the vagina. Soaps, bubble baths and shampoos can strip natural oils from the membranes that protect the vaginal walls.
- Use a condom when there's risk of a sexually transmitted disease.
- Wear underwear that's made from cotton rather than polyester. Cotton breathes more and allows the vagina to stay dry and cool.
- Sleep without underwear to allow adequate ventilation.
- Try using a less absorbent tampon or pads if vaginal dryness is a problem.

SELF-CARE

A burning or stinging sensation during urination is a very common medical problem. It occurs most often in women, but can occur in men as well. Other symptoms may include frequent urination and blood in the urine.

Urinary discomfort is usually caused by an irritation in the lining of the urethra (the tube bringing urine outside the body) because of an infection. Other contributing factors include sexual intercourse, perfumed soaps and scratching. Young girls are especially prone to infections because their urethras are very short.

The most common urinary infections in women are caused by bacteria found in the feces. Bubble baths increase the risk of infection because they can wash away protective fluids that protect the lining of the urethra and cause irritation.

In males, painful urination may be traced to a urinary tract infection or a sexually transmitted disease. A less likely cause is an enlarged prostate.

An enlarged prostate may result in slight discomfort during urination, but is more commonly associated with difficulty in urination, dribbling or decreased force in urinary flow. You should consult your doctor if these symptoms are present. Painful urination with a discharge from the penis may indicate a sexually transmitted disease or a urinary tract infection; consult your doctor.

CONSULT YOUR DOCTOR IF:

- You have a sudden onset of frequent, painful urination or blood in your urine.
- Your urinary problem is present with a body temperature of 100 degrees F or above.
- You have pain in one side of the small of the back, which may indicate a kidney infection.
- If male, you have difficulty with urination (e.g., interrupted flow, dribbling, fullness after urination) or have discharge from the penis.
- Your problem doesn't go away after three days of HomeCare.

HOMECARE

If physician referral is not recommended at this time, try the following self-care procedures:

- Drink plenty of fluids: 10 full glasses of water per day.
- In addition to water, drink cranberry juice, which contains a natural substance that helps kill bacteria.
- Avoid caffeine drinks until problem has passed.

- Women should avoid bubble baths, perfumed soap and douches that may irritate the urethra.
- Women should wipe from front to back after a bowel movement.

- Drink plenty of fluids.
- Prevent sexually transmitted diseases. Avoid sexual contact if you're unsure about the person's health status. At the very least, use a condom if you or your partner's disease status is not known.

92

TENSION HEADACHES

Most headaches are caused by muscular tension in the scalp and surrounding muscles of the jaw, neck, shoulders and back. *For most people, tension headaches are a physical/emotional reaction to outside stressors such as personal or work problems, working in one position for an extended period (such as word processing) and being exposed to excessive noise. Headaches are also a common symptom of viral infections such as a cold or flu, or bacterial infections such as sinusitis.*

Except for headaches caused by infections, headache pain is best treated by reducing the pressure in your life. Though sometimes difficult, changing your perception and reaction to stress can give significant relief.

Periodic tension headaches are rarely an indication of other health problems, such as a brain tumor or hypertension. Brain tumors are usually accompanied by other symptoms such as paralysis and personality changes.

CONSULT YOUR DOCTOR IF:

- Your headache is associated with fever and stiffness in the neck. This may indicate meningitis.

- Your headache is associated with slurred speech, dizziness, or weakness in your arms and legs.

- Your headache is accompanied by vision problems.

- Your headaches become much worse and more frequent.

* Because of the risk of Reye's syndrome, aspirin should not be given to or used by children or teenagers who have or are suspected of having flu or chicken pox. Use acetaminophen.

HOMECARE

If physician referral is not recommended at this time, try the following self-care procedures:

- Learn a deep muscle relaxation technique. Refer to p.17.

- Drink alcohol in moderation or not at all.
- Avoid drinking too much caffeine.

- Aspirin, ibuprofen or acetaminophen for relieving headache pain. Use as directed.

- Apply a heating pad or warm washcloth to back of neck.
- A long, hot shower or bath, followed by a self-massage to the back of the neck, temples and forehead may help.

- Exercise regularly. Regular physical activity has been shown to reduce stress and muscular tension.

- Massage the neck muscles.
- Check your work posture.

SELF-CARE

It's estimated that 18 million people suffer from migraine headaches. *"Classic" migraines are characterized by throbbing pain, usually on one side of the head; other symptoms include nausea, vomiting or dizziness. Some people experience an aura prior to onset of the headache: they see "stars," flashes of light or blind spots.* Common or "simple" migraine headaches usually cause pain throughout the head and are not accompanied by an aura.

Migraine and the more painful cluster headache are called vascular headaches, because experts believe that they are caused by the blood vessels (vasculature) in the head contracting, then expanding (dilate)—causing pain to the nerve endings of the head. Recent studies have pointed to the lack of a brain chemical called serotonin as the cause of the abnormal expansion of the blood vessels in the head.

All vascular headaches can be precipitated by a variety of factors such as certain foods (e.g., nuts, chocolate and aged cheese), alcohol (especially red wine), menstrual periods, irregular or excessive sleeping patterns, excessive use of pain killers, tobacco, a number of prescription drugs, and withdrawal from caffeine and other drugs.

Cluster headaches produce excruciating pain around one eye and reoccur repetitively over days weeks or months, then disappear for a period of time, only to occur again.

94

CONSULT YOUR DOCTOR IF:

- You suffer from migraine or cluster headaches. Most people who have these headaches require professional assessment and treatment. Your doctor may recommend medication and other alternative treatments such as biofeedback.

- Common vascular headache continues after HomeCare has been tried for more than a week.

* Because of the risk of Reye's syndrome, aspirin should not be given to or used by children or teenagers who have or are suspected of having flu or chicken pox. Use acetaminophen.

HOMECARE

If physician referral is not recommended at this time, try the following self-care procedures:

- Get adequate levels of sleep and rest.
- When headache occurs, go to a quiet, darkened room; lie down and relax your body. Refer to p. 17.

- Drink plenty of water. Avoid alcohol and caffeine drinks.

- Avoid chocolate, aged cheese, red wine and food additives such as nitrates and monosodium glutamate, which may increase symptoms.

- Aspirin, acetaminophen and ibuprofen are helpful in relieving tension headache pain, but may not be effective in treating vascular headaches such as migraine.
- Follow directions carefully when using prescription drugs.

- Try to stay physically active.

- For all vascular headaches: get plenty of sleep and relaxation, eat right (beware of special foods and food additives, such as nitrates), manage stress, avoid alcohol and tobacco.

INSOMNIA

It's estimated that approximately 20 percent of adults suffer from chronic sleeplessness. Twice as many women as men experience insomnia, and up to one third of adults over age 60 complain of sleep problems.

Sleep disorders are a leading cause of physician visits. The consequences, such as fatigue, low energy and poor concentration, are a significant reason for reduced work performance and increased accidents. *Sleeplessness is rarely caused by a physical problem. Rather, habits such as using caffeine, exercising close to bedtime, napping during the day, or feeling stressed or excited all can disrupt sleep patterns. Also the "rebound" that can occur a few hours after drinking alcohol may make getting to sleep difficult or cause awakening shortly after getting to sleep.*

Perhaps the greatest health risk resulting from sleep problems is the chronic use of sleep aids such as antihistamines or sleeping pills. Reliance on sleep aids can create dependency and increased tolerance. This can produce a cycle of unnatural sleep patterns and more fatigue.

CONSULT YOUR DOCTOR IF:

- The HomeCare recommendations do not improve your sleep pattern after four weeks.

HOMECARE

If physician referral is not recommended at this time, try the following self-care procedures:

- Avoid drinking alcohol and caffeine-containing drinks such as coffee, tea and colas.
- Don't use alcohol as a sleep aid.

- Associate your bed and bedroom with sleeping only.
- Practice a relaxation exercise. See p. 17.

- A hot bath or warm shower promotes muscle relaxation.

- Eating starches such as pasta can help promote relaxation and drowsiness. However, don't overdo it.
- Warm milk can also help you become drowsy.

- Avoid heavy exercise in the late evening. Exercise earlier in the day.

- If you can't sleep, get up and read in a chair until you feel drowsy.
- Avoid using sleep aids such as sedatives and antihistamines.

SELF-CARE

Everyone has their ups and downs. But if you find that you are frequently down or when you are down, that it seriously interferes with your usual activities, depression may be a likely diagnosis. In most cases, depression is a reaction to a major life event, such as the death of a loved one, separation, divorce or loss of a job. It can also be caused by interactions between various drugs, especially among the elderly. Chronic drinking of alcohol, even in moderate amounts, can cause or worsen depression. Also, any stimulant (including caffeine) can cause depression during withdrawal.

Depression can be mild to severe. Many depressed people describe their condition as *"living in a fog of depression."* They have limited interest in the activities of daily living. *Other symptoms include fatigue, lack of concentration, boredom, hopelessness, sleeping problems, pessimism, loss of sex drive, isolation and suicidal thoughts.*

SEEK PROFESSIONAL HELP IF:

- You have any thoughts of suicide. Call a suicide prevention hotline, found in the local white pages, or seek professional help through your doctor, local mental health clinic or clergy.

- You desire professional help in discussing your problem. Ask your doctor for a referral or contact your local mental health center or company employee assistance program.

96

HOMECARE

If physician referral is not recommended at this time, try the following self-care procedures:

- Have a confidant. Talk it out with a friend or family members. Don't be afraid to share your feelings with someone you trust.
- Try to focus on the positive aspects of life, rather than just problems.

- Avoid mood-altering drugs, especially illicit drugs such as marijuana or cocaine.
- Use prescription drugs only as directed.

- Avoid the use of alcohol in coping with your mood.

- Be active. Regular physical activity has been shown to help prevent and reduce mild depression in adults.

- Learning a relaxation technique can help reduce tension. See p. 17.

- Overeating and weight gain can be a common problem with depression. Avoid overeating and snacking. Eat well-balanced meals.

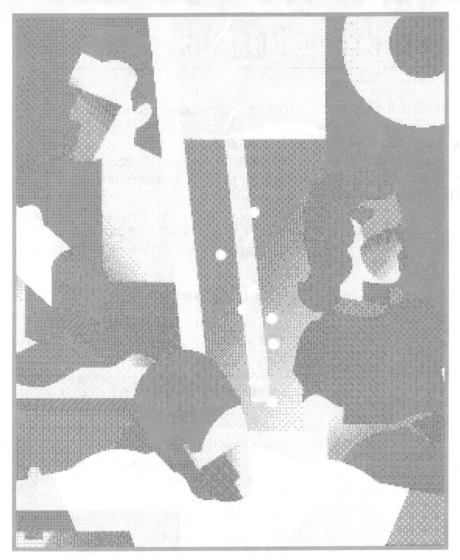

Special Health Issues

By Using This Section You Will:

• Learn about major health problems that are influenced by life-style choices.

• Learn how to prevent or manage such conditions as high blood pressure, high cholesterol and diabetes.

• Learn how to reduce the risk of premature labor and increase your chances of having a healthy baby.

• Learn how to protect your back and how to manage back pain.

• Learn the facts on AIDS and how to prevent its transmission.

Blood pressure is the amount of force blood exerts against artery walls as it flows through them. It is measured and recorded as two numbers: systolic pressure, the peak force when the heart beats (contracts); and diastolic pressure, the force against the artery walls when the heart is between beats.

"Normal" blood pressure traditionally has been defined as 120/80 mmHg (systolic pressure is the upper number; diastolic pressure is the lower number). Recently, however, the American Heart Association, working with the National High Blood Pressure Education Program, has modified the definition of acceptable blood pressure as below 130/85 mmHg. The lower the numbers, the lower your risk within reason. Blood pressure of 120/80 mmHg is still considered optimal.

People whose blood pressure is 140/90 or higher are considered to have high blood pressure, or hypertension, and should take steps to manage it. People who are at the "high normal range"—a systolic reading of 130 to 139 or a diastolic reading of 85 to 89—should also attempt to lower their blood pressure through behavior change. (See Ideas That Work for recommendations on managing high blood pressure.)

"Essential hypertension," where the cause cannot be determined, accounts for 90 percent of hypertension cases. The remaining 10 percent are caused by such conditions as kidney disease and tumors. Left untreated, high blood pressure increases the risk of stroke, heart disease, kidney failure and blindness.

Risk factors for high blood pressure include previous family history; gender (affects more males than females); race (affects African-Americans more than other ethnic groups); being overweight; high alcohol consumption; a sedentary lifestyle; uncontrolled stress; and excessive sodium (salt) consumption.

Blood pressure is easily measured through a pressure cuff, gauge and stethoscope or computerized instrument. It's recommended that you have your blood pressure measured once a year by a health professional. Home test kits can be purchased for home monitoring. The American Red Cross or your health care provider can teach you the proper way to measure your blood pressure.

IDEAS THAT WORK:

- **Prevention is the key.** Reduce your risk of developing hypertension with the following self-care practices: maintain your ideal weight; exercise three to five times per week; avoid eating prepared foods that are high in sodium; throw away the salt shaker; eat foods rich in potassium (e.g., bananas, oranges, potatoes and green vegetables) and calcium (e.g., low-fat milk and yogurt). If you smoke, try to quit. If you already have high blood pressure, the same strategies are recommended to manage and reduce it.

- **Follow your doctor's recommendations.** In general, if you have been diagnosed with hypertension, your doctor will not only recommend lifestyle changes (see above), but will also put you on a medication schedule. Your treatment usually is "stepped." With a stepped care plan, you begin by taking a small dose of a specific anti-hypertensive drug or drugs. You and your doctor carefully monitor blood pressure changes and any side effects. Standard hypertensive drugs include diuretics (which increase urination), beta blockers, calcium channel blockers, alpha blockers and angiotensin-converting-enzyme inhibitors (ACE).

• **Stick to it.** Don't change your treatment schedule without your doctor's prior approval. Be sure to take your medication as prescribed. Tell your doctor about any side effects, such as headaches, fatigue, and extra or skipped heart beats.

RESOURCES:

Your doctor

The American Red Cross. Check your phone directory for the chapter nearest you.

American Heart Association. Check your phone directory for the chapter nearest you.

SPECIAL ISSUES

Normally, the body breaks down the components of foods (carbohydrates, fats and protein) into glucose, which the body then uses as an energy supply. In a person with diabetes, the hormone that helps change glucose into energy—called insulin—is either *underproduced* or is *prevented* from working as it should. In either case, glucose levels in the blood rise to unacceptable levels. Persons with diabetes are at increased risk for damage to the blood vessels, kidneys, eyes and nervous system. People with insulin-dependent diabetes mellitus (IDDM) run the added risk of suffering a diabetic coma if their condition is left untreated.

There are two kinds of diabetes mellitus:

(1) **Insulin-dependent diabetes mellitus (IDDM)** may be an autoimmune disorder, where the body accidentally attacks the insulin-producing cells found in the pancreas. Also known as Type 1 diabetes, IDDM develops during childhood or young adulthood. Treatment includes daily injections of insulin or the use of an insulin pump to keep blood sugar levels under control; combined with a modified diet, moderate exercise and regular monitoring of blood sugar.

(2) **Noninsulin-dependent diabetes mellitis (NIDDM)** (or Type II diabetes) usually develops in people over 40 years of age. NIDDM, also called adult-onset diabetes, is strongly associated with obesity. Excess fat is believed to interfere with insulin's role in changing glucose to energy. People with NIDDM generally don't have to take insulin. Treatment includes a carefully planned diet, weight loss, moderate exercise, regular monitoring of blood sugar, and medication in some cases.

Common symptoms of diabetes include frequent urination, excessive thirst, weight loss, blurred vision, fatigue and loss of muscular coordination.

Testing for diabetes can be done by measuring sugar levels in the blood or the urine. The glucose tolerance test is among the most reliable: it measures blood sugar levels before and after the person drinks a specific dose of liquid glucose.

IDEAS THAT WORK:

- **Know the signs.** Be aware of the symptoms of diabetes, listed above. Consult your doctor if these symptoms begin and seem to persist or get worse over a few days.

- **Stick to your treatment.** Watch your diet, exercise regularly and monitor your blood glucose levels carefully. If you have IDDM, be sure to follow your insulin injection schedule. Know what is considered a normal blood sugar range and what needs to be reported to your doctor.

- **Watch your weight.** Help prevent NIDDM by staying within your ideal weight. Try to lose body fat if you are obese. Refer to p. 13, Weight Management.

- **Find support.** Because it requires daily maintenance over a lifetime, diabetes can be a difficult condition to cope with. Your local chapter of the American Diabetes Association can provide you with advice and resources.

RESOURCES:

American Diabetes Association
1660 Duke Street
Alexandria, VA 22313
(703) 549-1500 or your local chapter

CHOLESTEROL

Cholesterol is a waxy substance found in the tissue and blood stream of the body that is critical for maintaining healthy cell function. Our bodies manufacture cholesterol, and we also get it from eating certain foods, especially saturated fats. Within the body, cholesterol is transported through the blood stream by being attached to protein packages called lipoproteins. The two main lipoproteins are low-density lipoproteins (LDLs) and high-density lipoproteins (HDLs). HDLs are called the "good cholesterol," since they act as "garbage men" that prevent cholesterol from binding to the inner linings of blood vessels. The action of HDLs helps prevent the development of atherosclerosis, the major culprit in clogged arteries, leading to coronary artery disease and stroke. LDLs, on the other hand, are considered the "bad cholesterol" because high levels of LDLs in the body promote the development of atherosclerosis.

HOW IS CHOLESTEROL MEASURED?

Cholesterol is measured through blood analysis. First, a sample of blood is taken, either through a simple finger prick or by drawing blood from a vein. The sample is analyzed for total cholesterol and, if the need exists and the equipment is available, for LDLs and HDLs.

Cholesterol is measured in milligrams per deciliter (mg/dl). The chart below summarizes generally accepted values.

One way to measure heart disease risk is by computing the ratio of your total cholesterol level to HDL level; the higher the ratio, the greater the risk. (Example: 200 mg/dl total cholesterol divided by 45 mg/dl HDL gives a ratio of 4.4:1). *An acceptable ratio is 4.5:1 or lower.*

IDEAS THAT WORK:

- **Restrict your total intake of saturated fats.** Limit such foods as butter, hard cheeses, meat fat, and coconut, palm and hydrogenated vegetable oils. Replace saturated fats with monounsaturated fats found in olive and canola oils. Read food labels carefully. Try to keep your total intake of fats below 30 percent of daily calories and total intake of cholesterol below 300 mg.

- **Keep moving.** Increase your daily physical activity through aerobic exercise such as

TYPE	DESIRED LEVELS	MODERATE RISK	HIGH RISK
TOTAL CHOLESTEROL	Below 200 mg/dl	200 mg/dl to 239 mg/dl	240 mg/dl and higher
HDL	Above 60 mg/dl	35 to 59 mg/dl	Below 35 mg/dl
LDL	Below 130 mg/dl	130 to 159 mg/dl	Above 160 mg/dl

brisk walking, jogging, cycling and swimming. Regular physical activity increases the level of HDL, the good cholesterol, in your body.

- **Bulk up.** Increase your intake of soluble fiber, found in oat bran, apples, legumes and other vegetables. A good guideline is to try to eat a minimum of five servings of fruits and vegetables daily. Refer to p. 10.

- **Maintain your ideal weight.** Obese people have been found to have lower HDL concentrations and higher levels of LDL.

- **Learn to manage stress.** Some studies have shown that people who exhibit so-called "Type A" personality traits, such as free-floating hostility, extreme competitiveness, time urgency and impatience, have a higher rate of heart disease.

- **Follow your physician's advice.** Individuals who have cholesterol readings over 240 mg/dl may be advised by their physician to take a cholesterol-lowering medication, combined with practicing the life-style practices listed above.

- **Give me an "E"!** Taking a daily supplement of vitamin E (400 International Units) may help reduce the effectiveness of LDL cholesterol (the bad cholesterol) in damaging the artery walls. However, this *does not replace* the other strategies listed above in controlling your cholesterol.

- **Watch your numbers.** Experts recommend that all adults have their total cholesterol and HDL measured at least once and total cholesterol measured every three to five years thereafter.

If you have a family history of heart attack before age 50 or exhibit other risk factors such as diabetes, high blood pressure, obesity, smoking and a sedentary lifestyle, you should have total cholesterol and HDLs measured each time your doctor recommends cholestrol testing. Otherwise, if your total cholesterol is below 200 mg/dl, you have no family history of early heart disease or other coronary risk factors, you may not need to have your HDL and LDL levels measured regularly.

RESOURCES:

Your primary care physician.

Your local chapter of the American Heart Association. Check the white pages of your phone book.

ALCOHOL USE

Since the beginning of civilization, alcohol has been used for religious rituals and celebrations by rich and poor alike.

Classified as a depressant, alcohol is immediately absorbed through the stomach and affects every cell in the body. The brain, kidneys and lungs are especially affected by alcohol consumption.

How your body reacts to alcohol depends on a number of factors:

• **Dosage:** The higher the alcohol concentration, the faster the blood alcohol level will increase.

• **Drinking rate:** The more drinks taken within an hour, the faster the blood alcohol level will rise. The liver can normally metabolize one drink per hour with limited physical and mental effects on the user.

• **Alcohol and food:** Eating a meal will slow the absorption of alcohol through the stomach, whereas drinking on an empty stomach will accelerate absorption.

• **Alcohol tolerance:** Since alcoholics burn alcohol at a faster rate than non-alcoholics do, they need more alcohol to get the same effects.

• **Body weight:** Usually the greater the body weight, the more alcohol is needed for a person to become intoxicated. However, even amounts of alcohol that are perceived as modest (e.g., three beers within an hour for a 180 pound person), can significantly impair judgment and motor skills such as driving a car. In fact, a 180

What's Your Attitude About Alcohol?

The following self-test is designed to assess your attitudes and behaviors regarding alcohol.

How many of these statements do you agree with?

❏ I use alcohol to feel good.

❏ I often drink by myself.

❏ I use alcohol to forget my problems.

❏ As long as nobody gets hurt, it's nobody's business how much I drink.

❏ I drink and drive.

❏ I need a drink first thing in the morning.

❏ I often wake up from a heavy drinking session and don't remember where I was or what went on before I passed out.

❏ I have frequent hangovers after I drink.

❏ I like to boast about my ability to "tie one on."

❏ I feel I need to sneak a drink in order to calm my nerves.

❏ I have been told I have a drinking problem.

❏ I have been arrested for D.W.I. (Driving While Under the Influence).

❏ I have been warned by my supervisor about my drinking.

❏ I can't enjoy a social function unless alcohol is served.

❏ My drinking behavior leads to arguments with family members.

❏ I have become violent toward my family or others while under the influence of alcohol.

❏ I have felt angered and annoyed when someone criticized my drinking.

❏ I often feel guilty or embarrassed about my drinking behavior once I'm sober.

❏ I feel I have a drinking problem, but I refuse to get help.

What does this quiz mean?

If you found you agreed with one or more of these statements, you may have a problem with alcohol. It's recommended that you seek professional assistance. Start with your company or union employee assistance program, if available, or refer to the resources on p. 124.

pound person who drinks three beers in one hour would have a blood alcohol level of .05, which in many states is grounds for being arrested for "driving while under the influence" (D.W.I.).

Three Kinds Of Drinkers:

Millions of Americans are social drinkers: their use of alcohol is responsible and not habitual. When it comes to drinking, they can take it or leave it.

Why a person becomes a problem drinker or alcoholic is still debated. Problem drinkers are those individuals whose use of alcohol interferes with their interpersonal relationships, health and well-being. They also put themselves and others in danger due to their risky behaviors, e.g., driving while under the influence.

Alcoholics are individuals whose use of alcohol has gone out of control. On any particular day when they take their first drink, they cannot predict whether they will be able to stop before becoming drunk or passing out. They have developed a psychological and sometimes a physical dependence on alcohol. Alcoholics can suffer withdrawal symptoms such as DTs (delirium tremens) or severe alcohol poisoning. Both conditions can be fatal.

Getting Help...
The First Step To Recovery:

The first and most critical step in treating alcohol dependency is getting the problem drinker to admit that a serious problem exists and that change cannot happen without the help of others.

Another critical step in the treatment process is getting the problem drinker to realize that he or she has a behavioral problem as well as a medical condition. It's not uncommon to hear about

an alcoholic receiving a liver transplant, only to go back to the bottle after surgery. The bottom line: Unless a problem drinker can admit that he or she has a problem with alcohol, and begin to adopt more positive coping skills, long-term recovery is questionable.

Start With These Resources For Help:

- If available, your employee assistance program
- Local or national alcohol hotlines
- Local community alcohol rehabilitation centers (listed in the yellow pages)
- Anonymous groups; e.g., Alcoholics Anonymous (listed in the white pages)
- Your personal physician
- Your priest, minister or rabbi

How To Help A Person With A Drinking Problem:

It's very difficult to confront someone about his or her drinking, especially if there is a risk of mental and physical abuse. Friends, coworkers and "drinking buddies" are often reluctant to confront the person; they become "enablers" by ignoring or denying the problem and encouraging it to continue. The more drinking behavior a person is exposed to, the more difficult it is for him or her to recognize normal behavior. This may be one of the reasons children of alcoholics will marry alcoholics; in the dating process they don't notice that the partner's drinking is abnormal.

IDEAS THAT WORK: Getting Involved

If you wish to help an individual who has a serious drinking problem, be prepared for an up-hill climb. It's not easy. In the short term you may be perceived as the enemy, especially if you persist. Here are some suggestions:

- **Learn about the problem.** Contact such resources as your company employee assistance program, alcohol rehabilitation center and Alcoholics Anonymous (AA).

- **Confront the person when he or she is sober.**

- **Focus on behavior only.** Focus on how the person's drinking affects his or her behavior in relation to work, family and friends. Be objective and stick to the facts: "When you were drunk last night, you threw a shoe at me. Do you remember that happening?"

- **Expect denial.** It's common for problem drinkers to deny their problem until some event forces them to face it.

- **Ease up.** If your first efforts fail to convince the person to seek help, ease up on your feedback. There will be another opportunity.

- **Offer support.** Reinforce your interest in supporting the problem drinker when he or she decides to quit.

- **Avoid abuse.** Never tolerate mental or physical abuse, either as a recipient or observer. Get help before someone really gets hurt.

- **You may want to try the intervention method.** In an intervention, a trained alcohol counselor joins family, friends and sometimes coworkers to confront the person about his or her drinking behavior. The goal of an intervention is to get the person to realize that he or she has a problem and to agree immediately to rehabilitation.

- **Expect denial when confronting the individual.** It's common for alcohol abusers to deny their problem until the bitter end. In fact, the threat of job loss may be the only thing that pushes a person to seek help; without income there's no money to pay for alcohol.

Working Toward Sobriety:

Experts agree that staying sober is a lifelong commitment. Treatment depends on each person's situation, and can range from a "lay network" such as Alcoholics Anonymous (AA) to outpatient or inpatient care using an intensive medical and behavioral approach.

- **Inpatient programs.** An in-house treatment program through a local hospital or residential treatment center usually is recommended if the person with an alcohol problem has immediate medical needs (overdose, withdrawal) or psychological needs (suicidal thoughts) that place him or her in danger. **Warning:** Because of the high cost of residential alcohol rehabilitation programs (up to $15,000 for a 12-day stay), make sure that your medical benefit program approves treatment before being admitted for a nonemergency. Discuss other treatment options such as outpatient care.

- **Outpatient programs.** These community-based programs combine one-on-one counseling sessions and group sessions. Usually patients are referred to a local AA group for ongoing support and assistance.

- **Alcoholics Anonymous.** Many alcoholics have been successful in staying sober through AA. This self-help approach guides a person through 12 carefully designed steps to becoming and remaining sober. In AA, there is continual emphasis on the need for recovering alcoholics to support and help one another in maintaining sobriety. Studies show that the longer people attend AA, the longer they stay sober.

• **Family assistance.** There are many support organizations and services that can assist family members in coping with a problem drinker.The first resource, if available, should be your company or union employee assistance program. Other organizations such as Al-Anon or Alateen can assist family members in dealing with the stresses of living with an alcoholic. MADD (Mothers Against Drunk Driving) sponsors programs against drunk driving (e.g., designated driver programs) and local support groups for families who have lost family members because of a drunk driver.

Remember, if you or someone you know has a drinking problem, help is available. Please seek it now!

RESOURCES:

Your company or union employee assistance program, if available.

Alcoholics Anonymous (AA)
General Service Office
P.O. Box 459, Grand Central Station
New York, NY 10163;
(212) 870-3400

Al-Anon/Alateen
Family Group Headquarters
P.O. Box 862, Midtown Station
New York, NY 10018-0862; (212) 302-7240

National Institute on Alcohol Abuse and Alcoholism (NIAAA)
Parklawn Building,
5600 Fishers Lane
Rockville, MD 20857; (301) 443-3860

Mothers Against Drunk Driving:
(800) 438-6233

Check your phone book's white pages for AA and Al-Anon groups near you.

Turn on the television or read the newspaper, and the impact of drugs on our society will be very evident. But contrary to what you may hear or see, drug abuse is not limited to the crack houses of the inner city or the glamorous "jet set." In fact, you may be working or living with a person who has a drug problem.Victims of drug abuse include:

- *The users themselves. Drug abuse leads to physical and/or psychological addiction. If people share needles for intravenous drug use, they put themselves and sexual partners at risk of HIV or hepatitis infection.*

- *The family. Families of drug users may suffer neglect, and physical and mental abuse. Pregnant women who use drugs such as heroin and cocaine place their unborn children at a greater risk for birth defects and infectious disease.*

- *Coworkers. Employees who work with a drug abuser may be victims of unsafe work practices and the abuser's unreliable job performance.*

- *Companies. Employees who abuse drugs cost companies money through increased health and disability claims, defective products and a damaged reputation in the marketplace.*

- *Society. Consumers may suffer from defective products or services; people who use public transportation are at risk from operators who may use drugs on the job. Drug abuse costs taxpayers billions of dollars for treatment and law enforcement—money that could be spent on education, job training and other needed services.*

How Do Drugs Work?

Drugs that alter the chemistry of the brain and nervous system are called psychoactive agents. A psychoactive agent can act as a stimulant, a depressant or a hallucinogen. Psychoactive substances are not limited to illegal "street drugs" such as cocaine, heroin and marijuana, but also include prescription and over-the-counter medications, as well as the most widely used drugs: alcohol, nicotine and caffeine. Each drug has a unique effect on the mind and body of the user, and can lead to a physical and/or psychological dependence.

• **Stimulants**

Stimulants, or "uppers," raise the metabolism of the user. People use stimulants to stay alert, to get a rapid surge of energy and to lose weight. "Household" stimulants include coffee, tea, cola drinks and tobacco: caffeine and nicotine both stimulate the central nervous system. Commonly used stimulants that are "controlled substances" (drugs that are strictly controlled or banned by federal laws) include cocaine and its highly addictive derivative, crack; amphetamines; and methamphetamine (speed).

• **Depressants**

Commonly known as "downers," depressants slow down the activity of the central nervous system and alter people's perception of the outside world by narrowing their field of focus. Users commonly become withdrawn and "spaced out." Depressants include sedatives, sleep aids and painkillers.

Alcohol is the most widely used depressant, although many people think it's a stimulant since it decreases people's inhibitions (see p. 103). Controlled substances that are classified as depressants include barbiturates; narcotic agents such as heroin, morphine, opium and codeine; and synthetic drugs such as *Percodan*, *Demerol* and *Darvon*.

• Hallucinogens

Hallucinogens are chemical agents that alter a person's sense of reality. "Tripping" is the common term used to describe the effect of hallucinogens in enhancing and intensifying perception. LSD, mescaline, peyote and magic mushrooms are substances that are normally ingested to produce hallucinogenic effects. An especially dangerous hallucinogen is PCP, or "Angel Dust," which often produces violent and unpredictable behavior in users. PCP is usually combined with marijuana or other leafy substances such as oregano or parsley, rolled in a cigarette and smoked.

• Cannabis

Cannabis products are taken from the leaves of the hemp plant and are usually sold as marijuana (grass), hashish (hash), hashish oil or the chemical derivative THC (tetrahydrocannabinol). Usually smoked, cannabis products relax the user and create a mild sense of euphoria. In specific cases, cannabis has been prescribed to cancer patients to counteract the effects of chemotherapy.

Long-term use of cannabis has been linked to lung disease and a weakening of the immune system. Cannabis also affects memory, judgment, coordination and other sensory motor skills, and can impair a person's ability to drive and operate machinery.

Do You Need Help?

Our message is simple: The use of illicit or other drugs is the quickest way to destroy your career and personal life. Unfortunately, many abusers wait to get help until their problem has compromised their life to such an extent that they have lost everything they value. If you think you have a drug problem, it's important to get help right away.

Getting Help... The First Step To Recovery:

The first step to overcoming a dependence on drugs is admitting that a problem exists and that change can't happen without the help of others. Most drug abusers say that this first step is the most difficult. Rehabilitation programs have up to a 70 percent success rate, and can help the person in recovery realize that he or she doesn't need drugs to cope or for instant gratification.

The following are resources that can provide professional support for drug treatment and recovery:

• If available, your company employee assistance program

• Local or national drug hotlines

• Anonymous Groups; e.g., Narcotics Anonymous (listed in the white pages)

• Local community drug rehabilitation centers (listed in the yellow pages)

• Your personal physician

• Your priest, minister or rabbi

Recognizing Substance Abuse In Others:

It's common for many people to attribute a person's erratic behavior to anything but drug abuse, especially if the individual is a professional or celebrity. When a person has a drug problem, he or she is usually sending out signals for help. Some signs are hard to detect, while others are more obvious. The following are indications that a person may have a drug problem:

• Increased absences or tardiness at work

- Poor health habits
- Physical symptoms such as red eyes and sleepiness (marijuana); a chronic runny nose and bad breath (cocaine); scars or needle marks and constricted pupils that don't respond to light (heroin)
- Presence of drug paraphernalia such as roach clips, pipes, rolling papers, syringes, razor blades and straws
- Behavioral symptoms such as confusion, hyperactivity, excitability, mood swings and explosive bouts of anger
- Taking extended breaks or being absent from workstation
- Complaints about money; requests to borrow money from coworkers, friends or family
- Strained or abusive relationships with co-workers, friends or family.

How to Help Drug Abusers Quit:

It's very difficult to confront someone about their drug use. Family members and friends often become "enablers": they enable the drug user to continue his or her behavior by ignoring, denying or covering up the problem.

If you suspect that someone you know and care about has a drug problem, but don't know how to address the problem, try the following strategies:

- Learn about the problem by contacting such resources as your company employee assistance program, local drug rehabilitation center or drug hotline. The professional will advise you how to communicate your concerns to the drug user and will provide you with possible options for referral.
- You may want to try the intervention method. In an intervention, a trained drug counselor joins family, friends and sometimes co-workers to confront the drug user about his or her behavior. The goal of an intervention is to get the person to realize that he or she has a problem and to agree immediately to rehabilitation.
- Expect denial when confronting the individual. It's common for drug users to deny their problem until the bitter end. In fact, the threat of job loss may be the only thing that pushes a person to seek help; without income there's no money to pay for drugs.
- If your efforts fail to convince the person to seek help, be persistent in voicing your disapproval of the individual's behavior, but share your interest in supporting a decision to quit. Avoid becoming or remaining an enabler.

Working Through The Treatment Process:

Experts agree that recovery from drug dependence is a lifelong challenge. Although treatment depends on each person's individual needs and situation, the rehabilitation process usually follows these basic steps:

- Assessment. An assessment is conducted to evaluate the person's physical and psychological needs. The assessment usually is done by a team of health professionals, such as a physician and a mental health professional specializing in addictions. The team recommends a treatment plan based on the results of the evaluation.
- Determining treatment. Depending on the severity of the problem, health professionals may advise an in-house treatment program

in a local hospital or residential treatment center. In-house programs usually are recommended if the person has immediate medical needs (overdose, withdrawal) or psychological needs (threat of suicide) that place him or her in danger.

Warning: Because of the high costs of residential drug rehabilitation programs (up to $15,000 for a 12-day stay), make sure that your health insurance plan approves treatment before you are committed for a nonemergency. Check other options, such as outpatient care.

• **Most drug treatment is done on an outpatient basis.** Some outpatient programs require the person to attend an immersion program, in which he or she attends all-day sessions for two to four weeks while living at home. The program usually combines one-on-one counseling, therapist-led group sessions and instruction in appropriate self-care skills.

• **Transitions.** The recovering person usually progresses from professionally led group therapy sessions to community-based self-help groups such as Narcotics Anonymous. Participants often follow a 12-Step Program, which relies heavily on group support and commitment to lifelong recovery.

• Follow-up. The therapist or physician will schedule periodic visits to assess the person's progress and his or her need for further therapy.

RESOURCES:

Your company employee assistance program, if available.

National Clearinghouse for Alcohol and Drug Information
P.O. Box 2345
Rockville, MD 20847
(800) 729-6686

American Council for Drug Education
204 Monroe Street, Suite 110
Rockville, MD 20850
(301) 294-0600

National Cocaine Hotline: (800) COCAINE

National Institute on Drug Abuse Hotline: (800) 662-HELP

Narcotics Anonymous. Check your phone directory's white pages.

PLANNING YOUR PREGNANCY

The chart below is designed to help women who are planning to have a baby understand the potential risks of certain behaviors and the potential effects on the health of the baby and the mother. *The more high-risk behaviors that you plan to continue during your pregnancy, the greater your chances of premature labor or other serious problems.*

If you have any of the risk factors described below, discuss them with your doctor before conception. If you find out that you're pregnant and have any of these risk factors, see your doctor as soon as possible to discuss your care plan. The right-hand column (Ideas That Work) provides you with additional assistance. *However, these ideas are not a substitute for appropriate medical supervision.*

RISK FACTORS	CONSEQUENCES OF CONTINUING OR NOT CONTROLLING RISK FACTORS	IDEAS THAT WORK
• **Smoking** ❑ Smoking while pregnant ❑ Continued exposure to smoke-filled rooms	**For You:** • Miscarriage • Premature delivery **For Your Baby:** • Low birthweight • SIDS (Sudden Infant Death Syndrome)	• Stop smoking before you're pregnant. • Enroll in a stop-smoking program. • Avoid smoke-filled areas. • Refer to Resources.
• **Alcohol** ❑ Drinking 3-5 or more drinks a day before conception ❑ Drinking alcohol while pregnant	**For You:** • Miscarriage • Premature delivery • Liver problems • Accidents (e.g., drunken driving) • Alcoholism **For Your Baby:** • FAS (Fetal Alcohol Syndrome), leading to emotional and learning problems • Birth defects, mental retardation • Low birthweight • Increased death rate	• Don't drink while you're trying to get pregnant. • Don't drink alcohol during pregnancy or while nursing your baby. • If you have a drinking problem, seek help. See Alcohol Use, p. 103.
• **Drug Use** ❑ Using illegal drugs (crack, cocaine, heroin, marijuana) ❑ Using prescription or over-the-counter drugs during pregnancy without physician's approval	**For You:** • Miscarriage • Conception problems (cocaine and marijuana) • AIDS or hepatitis from IV drug use • Premature delivery **For Your Baby:** • Low birthweight • Addiction • AIDS or hepatitis virus from mother	• Abstain from all illegal drugs. • Get help if you have a drug problem *before* you become pregnant. • If you use any prescription or over-the-counter drugs (e.g., antihistamines), make sure your doctor approves their use. • Refer to Drug Abuse, p. 107.

S P E C I A L   I S S U E S

RISK FACTORS	CONSEQUENCES OF CONTINUING OR NOT CONTROLLING RISK FACTORS	IDEAS THAT WORK
• Obesity ❑ Being 20% or more over ideal weight	**For You:** • High blood pressure • Diabetes • Slow healing of incisions **For Your Baby:** • Delivery problems from heavier-than-average baby	• Achieve an acceptable weight before you become pregnant. • Follow your doctor's recommendations on proper nutrition and exercise. • Keep your weight gain within 35 pounds during your pregnancy. • Refer to p.13.
• Eating Disorders ❑ Always on a diet ❑ Binge eating, followed by forced vomiting (bulimia) ❑ Never feel thin enough ❑ Extremely concerned about weight gain during pregnancy	**For You:** • Premature delivery • Anemia **For Your Baby:** • Impaired growth and development • Low birthweight • Birth defects • Increased death rate	• Expect to gain between 25 to 35 pounds during your pregnancy. • Eat balanced meals. • Don't try to lose weight during pregnancy. • Don't take diet pills. • If you have an eating disorder, e.g., bulimia or anorexia, seek assistance. • Refer to Resources.
• Sexually Transmitted Diseases (STDs) ❑ Have already or may have been exposed to herpes, gonorrhea, syphilis, chlamydia HIV (AIDS virus) or hepatitis.	**For You:** • Miscarriage • Premature delivery • Complications during delivery • AIDS **For Your Baby:** • Birth defects • Increased risk of getting STD from mother (e.g., AIDS) • Eye infections (e.g., from herpes)	• If you think you already have or have been exposed to any STD, see your doctor *before* getting pregnant. • Avoid high-risk groups. Refer to p. 117.
• Age ❑ Are you age 35 or older or under age 18?	**For You:** • Miscarriage • Labor complications **For Your Baby:** • Increased risk for some birth defects, e.g., Down's syndrome if over age 35.	• If you have high blood pressure, diabetes or heart disease, see your doctor before becoming pregnant. • Get early and continued medical supervision. • Refer to Resources.
• Other ❑ You **are not** taking a daily supplement of folic acid.	**For Your Baby:** • Increased risk of neural tube defects, e.g., Spina bifida	• During pregnancy, women should take daily supplement of folic acid (0.4 mg.)

PREVENTING PRETERM LABOR

When a woman goes into labor three or more weeks before her baby is due, it is described as a preterm labor. If a woman has a premature baby, it increases the child's chances of having health problems because the baby's body is not well enough developed to live outside the mother's womb.

IDEAS THAT WORK:

- **Who is at risk?** You are at a greater risk for having a premature baby if you:

  - *Are pregnant with more than one child.*

  - *Had a premature baby previously.*

  - *Smoke, drink alcohol, misuse drugs.*

  - *Are a DES daughter. Your mother took hormones when pregnant with you.*

  - *Are younger than 18 years old or older than 35.*

  - *Are under a lot of stress and personal pressure.*

  - *Are bleeding from the vagina.*

  - *Have had two or more second trimester abortions or miscarriages.*

  - *Have had three or more urinary tract infections during this pregnancy.*

  - *If you have any of these conditions or other problems, discuss them with your doctor.*

- How to reduce the chance of a premature delivery.

  - *Review your risk factors before you try to conceive. See p. 111.*

  - *See a doctor as soon as you find out you're pregnant, and on a regular basis thereafter.*

  - *Stop smoking, drinking alcohol and using drugs. Check with your doctor before taking any medication.*

  - *Eat a well-balanced diet and gain the weight your doctor recommends.*

  - *Get enough rest.*

  - *Find support from friends and other people who can help when you are stressed or feel down.*

  - *Know the signs of labor and what to do when experiencing premature labor.*

  - *Be aware of what prenatal education services your insurance company, company or local hospital may sponsor. Do your own research.*

- Signs of premature labor include:

  - *Contraction of the uterus;*

  - *Menstrual-like cramps that come and go or don't go away;*

  - *Pelvic pressure: a feeling that the baby is pushing down; it may come and go;*

  - *A low, dull backache that comes and goes or doesn't go away;*

  - *Abdominal cramping with or without diarrhea;*

  - *Leakage or bleeding from the vagina.*

- If you show signs of premature labor, do the following:

  - *Lie down on your left side for an hour.*

  - *Drink two to three glasses of water or juice.*

  - *If the signs do not go away in one hour, or you have fluid leaking from your vagina, call your doctor or clinic immediately.*

Adapted and used with permission from *Baby Benefits*, Health Management Corporation, Richmond, Virginia.

RESOURCES:

Your Primary Care Physician

March of Dimes. Contact your local chapter.

Did you know that four out of five people experience some sort of back pain during their lifetime?

Back injuries can be caused by overexertion, poor posture, jarring from motor vehicles, slips and falls, stress, excessive body weight, and lack of exercise. The leading cause of back injuries is improper lifting techniques.

The following ideas and exercises will help you keep your back healthy and, if you have a back problem, will help you manage it. (*If you do have a back problem, consult with your doctor before you try any of the exercises on p. 116.*)

IDEAS THAT WORK:

• **Improve your backspring: stay active.**

- *Try to exercise three to five days per week, with aerobic activities such as brisk walking, swimming, cycling and jogging. See Walking, p. 8.*

- *Keep your stomach and lower back muscles strong. See p. 116.*

- *Warm up with simple stretches before you do lifting or twisting movements. See p. 116.*

• **Take off that extra weight, especially around your middle.** Maintain your ideal weight by cutting down on fatty foods and staying active. See Weight Management on p. 13.

• **Relax.** Learn and practice relaxation techniques to help prevent or reduce stress and tension. See p. 17.

• **Sleep on a firm mattress.** If your mattress is too soft, consider putting a sheet of plywood under it or purchasing an orthopedic mattress.

• **Reduce your load.** Avoid lifting and carrying loads that are too heavy, especially if the object is bulky and hard to keep close to your body. Lighten the load and take more trips, use a handcart or ask for help.

• **Take a break.** If you sit or stand for extended periods of time, take hourly stretch breaks.

• **Proper lifting:**

- *When you're carrying a load, turn your whole body in the direction you need to go. Avoid twisting or jerking movements.*

- *Stack material you're carrying in such a manner that your view is clear while you're carrying it.*

- *If the load to be lifted weighs more than 30 lbs., use two people to make the lift or use mechanical means (hoist, etc.).*

- *If the two-man load weighs more than 70 lbs., hand holds should be provided for accomplishing the lift.*

- *When two people carry a long object, they should hold it at the same level and on the same side of the body.*

- *Setting the load down is just as important as picking it up. Lower the load by bending your knees, keeping your back straight.*

- *Avoid strain when lifting by storing heavy objects at least 12 inches above the floor.*

- *Don't overreach or overstretch to reach objects stored overhead. This can result in strains or falls.*

- *Wear shoes with firm, slip-resistant soles.*

- *Never hurry or run when you're carrying a load.*

- *Use mechanical aids such as hand trucks if appropriate.*

- *When wearing gloves, make sure you have a firm grip before trying to lift.*

- *Consider wearing a lifting belt that supports the lower back.*

AIDS Facts

W ho hasn't heard of AIDS? AIDS, or acquired immune deficiency syndrome, is a disease that frightens most people. Anyone can get AIDS, but the chances are rare, unless you're involved in risky behaviors (see below) or are exposed to the virus accidentally.

Today, there is hardly anyone who doesn't know at least something about this tragic illness. However, knowing and understanding are often two vastly different things. Many people are afraid of AIDS and individuals infected with HIV (human immunodeficiency virus), the cause of AIDS, because they don't understand the facts.

Understanding what this disease is, how it's spread and who is at risk can reduce your risk of getting it. Having the right information can also help you show compassion and support for individuals you may know who have AIDS.

HIV causes AIDS and gradually damages the body's natural immune defenses against disease. It can also infect cells in the brain. People who have AIDS develop unusual, life-threatening illnesses that do not affect people with normal immune systems.

Most persons with HIV infection go through a series of stages:

• **Acute Primary Infection.** This stage usually lasts four to 12 weeks. The person experiences mono-like symptoms such as sore throat, fever, fatigue and swollen lymph glands. During this period, the body is producing antibodies, indicating it is trying to fight the infection. Antibodies are usually present within three months of infection. A blood test (Elisa) is used to detect HIV antibodies. A positive test (HIV positive) indicates the likelihood of HIV. A second more sensitive test is done to confirm the first. Infected persons can infect others. See below: *"How is the AIDS virus spread?"*

• **Latent Phase.** A period of 10 to 12 years during which the infected person has no symp-toms. However, the person is infectious and can transmit HIV. See *"How is the AIDS virus spread?"*

• **Active Phase.**

- *ARC: Some individuals develop a condition that is called "AIDS-related complex" (ARC). Symptoms include fever, feeling tired, loss of appetite, weight loss, diarrhea, night sweats, and swollen lymph nodes in the neck, armpits or groin. Persons can have ARC-related symptoms for weeks or years, die from complications or develop full-blown AIDS.*

- *AIDS: The severe end stage of the disease, with a variety of complications that further compromise the body's immune system. Two of the illnesses most often seen in AIDS patients are pneumocystis carinii pneumonia (a parasitic infection of the lungs) and Kaposi's sarcoma, a rare type of cancer.*

It's estimated that between one million and 1.5 million Americans are HIV positive and carry the virus in their bodies (this is in addition to those known to have AIDS). Many people who are more recently infected and are HIV positive show no signs of illness and do not know they carry the virus. However, they can spread it to others through sexual contact or contaminated blood products.

If a person tests positive for HIV through a special antibody test of the blood, it doesn't mean that the person has AIDS or will go on to get AIDS or an AIDS-related illness in the near future. It can take up to 10 years for someone to show symptoms of HIV infection and progress to AIDS. Though there is no cure, new treatments are becoming available that are helping individuals manage their condition, extend their lives and lead a more independent life.

WORK WITH THESE FACTS:

How is the AIDS virus spread?

• The virus is NOT spread through casual contact. The virus dies very quickly when it comes in contact with air or light.

AIDS Facts

- The virus IS spread through direct transmission to the bloodstream during unsafe (unprotected) sexual contact, through sharing needles, from contaminated blood products and by an HIV positive mother to her baby during birth.

- Casual kissing carries an extremely low risk; deep kissing (french kissing) hasn't been linked to transmittal of the virus, unless the infected person passes blood to the partner.

- You can't catch AIDS from donating blood. All needles used for blood donation are sterile and are never reused.

- AIDS has never been shown to be transmitted through insect bites.

- AIDS can't be spread by shaking hands, hugging or other forms of casual contact.

- Once outside the body, the AIDS virus dies quickly, so you can't catch it from drinking glasses, drinking fountains or toilet seats.

Who is at risk for catching AIDS?

- Individuals with the highest risk for carrying HIV have been homosexuals and bisexuals, intravenous drug users, male and female prostitutes and individuals who have sex or share needles with individuals from these high-risk groups. However, heterosexual risk is climbing. The World Health Organization reports that 90 percent of all new AIDS cases worldwide are from heterosexual contact.

- Anyone who has unprotected (unsafe) sex and who has not been in a mutually monogamous relationship for at least the last 10 years (HIV can exist for up to 10 years without symptoms) may have increased risk for getting AIDS.

- Anyone who has received blood transfusions before early 1985 is at risk. Since that time, all blood used for transfusions has been screened for HIV.

- Infants born to AIDS-infected mothers have a 20 to 30 percent chance of developing AIDS.

- People working in certain professions, such as police, firefighters, funeral home workers, emergency medical workers, dental personnel, prison staff and medical workers, who are routinely exposed to possible contaminated blood and body fluids, have a higher risk for contracting the disease, although the risk is small if proper precautions are followed.

How can I reduce my risk of catching AIDS?

- Do not have unsafe (unprotected) sex. If you do, make sure your partner is not infected. Otherwise, use a latex condom. For added protection, buy condoms that contain the spermicide nonoxynol-9 (condoms alone are not 100 percent effective against infection).

- Consider abstinence or a monogamous relationship with an uninfected partner when evaluating your own sexual behavior.

- If your job involves exposure to blood and body fluids, wear personal protective equipment such as gloves, masks, gowns and face shields. Make sure the equipment is the right type of material and is in good condition.

- Do not share needles if you are an IV drug user. Get some help to kick the habit.

RESOURCES:

Your doctor or primary health care provider

Your state or local health department: Check your phone directory for local listings.

AIDS toll-free hotline: (800) 342-AIDS

AIDS Education Office
American Red Cross
1730 D Street NW
Washington, DC 20006
(202) 434-4074

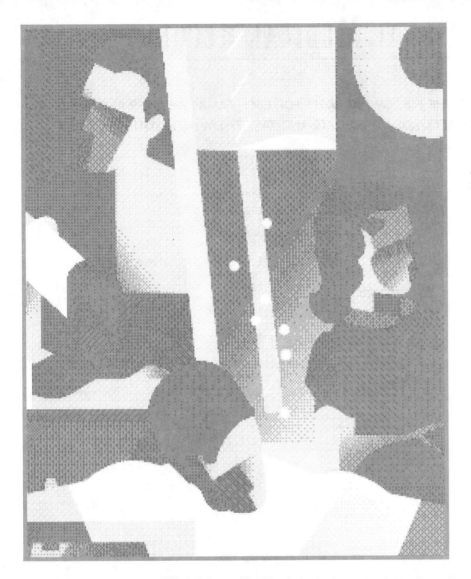

Appendix: Family Medical Records/Resources

BY USING THIS SECTION YOU WILL:
• Learn how to maintain a medical record-keeping system for you and your family.
• Learn how to record and track medication use for you and your family.

Personal Medical Record

Make a photocopy of the following pages for each family member and file in a safe place. Keep these records up-to-date and take them with you when you change doctors.

Family Member's Name: _____

Date of Birth: _____

Problems at Birth: _____

_____

Blood Type: _____   **Rh Factor:** _____

Childhood Diseases

Chicken Pox   Date _____
Measles   Date _____
Mumps   Date _____
Whooping Cough   Date _____
Rubella (German Measles) Date _____

Other Illnesses:

Illness: _____   Date: _____
Comments _____
_____

Illness: _____   Date: _____
Comments _____
_____

Illness: _____   Date: _____
Comments _____
_____

Illness: _____   Date: _____
Comments _____

Personal Medical Record

_____

ALLERGIES:

TYPE: _____   MEDICATION _____
ALLERGIC TO WHAT?   _____
                     _____
                     _____

TYPE: _____   MEDICATION _____
ALLERGIC TO WHAT?   _____
                     _____
                     _____

TYPE: _____   MEDICATION _____
ALLERGIC TO WHAT?   _____
                     _____
                     _____

HOSPITALIZATIONS:

REASON   _____   DATE _____ TO _____
DOCTOR   _____
HOSPITAL   _____
COMMENTS: _____
           _____
           _____

REASON   _____   DATE _____ TO _____
DOCTOR   _____
HOSPITAL   _____
COMMENTS: _____
           _____
           _____

PERSONAL IMMUNIZATION RECORD

FAMILY MEMBER'S NAME _____

DATE OF BIRTH _____

IMMUNIZATION	DATE	DOCTOR'S NAME	COMMENTS
Diptheria Pertussis Tetanus (DPT)	___ ___ ___ ___ ___	_____ _____ _____ _____ _____	_____ _____ _____ _____ _____
Adult Diptheria and Tetanus	___	_____	_____
Oral Polio (OPV)	___ ___ ___ ___ ___	_____ _____ _____ _____ _____	_____ _____ _____ _____ _____
Measles, Mumps and Rubella (MMR)	___ ___ ___	_____ _____ _____	_____ _____ _____
Hemophilus B	___ ___ ___	_____ _____ _____	_____ _____ _____
Influenza	___ ___ ___	_____ _____ _____	_____ _____ _____
Pneumococcal Pneumonia	___ ___	_____ _____	_____ _____
Hepatitis B	___ ___ ___	_____ _____ _____	_____ _____ _____
Other	___ ___	_____ _____	_____ _____

MEDICATION USE RECORD

MILY MEMBERS' NAME

ase make a copy of this page for each member of your family. Take this form with you when you visit the ctor. If a prescription and/or over-the-counter medication is recommended, have your doctor fill out the ormation below. **Be sure you understand the instructions. Do not change your treatment schedule less first consulting with your doctor. Keep this form in a safe place.**

Name of Drug? Date Prescribed? M.D.'s Name?	Used to Treat What Problem?	How Much?	How Many Times A Day? For How Long?	With Food Or On An Empty Stomach?	Fluids Recommended? Alcohol Prohibited?	Do Not Take With Other Drugs

INFORMED Resources

AIDS
National AIDS Information
Clearinghouse
P.O. Box 6003
Rockville, MD 20849-6003
(800) 458-5231

ALCOHOL
AA—Alcoholics Anonymous
P.O. Box 459, Grand Central
Station
New York, NY 10163
(212) 870-3400

Al-Anon/Alateen Family Group
Headquarters
P.O. Box 862, Midtown Station
New York, NY 10018-0862
(212) 302-7240

National Clearinghouse for
Alcohol and Drug Information
P.O. Box 2345
Rockville, MD 20847
(800) 729-6686

DRUG ABUSE
National Institute on Drug Abuse
(NIDA)
Parklawn Building, Room 9A53
5600 Fishers Lane
Rockville, MD 20857
(301) 443-0802

Cocaine Anonymous
3740 Overland Avenue, Suite H
Los Angeles, CA 90034
(213) 559-5833; (800) 347-8998
(meeting referrals)

Drugs Anonymous
P.O. Box 473
Ansonia Station
New York, NY 10023
(212) 874-0700

Narcotics Anonymous
P.O. Box 9999
Van Nuys, CA 91409
(818) 780-3951

EXERCISE/FITNESS
American College
of Sports Medicine
P.O. Box 1440
Indianapolis, IN 46206
(317) 637-9200

National Fitness Leaders
Association
14800 Conference Center Dr.
Chantilly, VA 22021
(703) 222-2520

President's Council on Physical
Fitness and Sports
450 5th Street, N.W. Suite 7103
Washington, DC 20001
(202) 272-3421

GENERAL HEALTH
American Cancer Society
90 Park Avenue
New York, NY 10016
(212) 599-3600
or (800) ACS-2345

American College of Preventive
Medicine
1015 15th Street NW, #403
Washington, DC 20005
(202) 789-0003

American Dental Association
211 East Chicago Avenue
Chicago, IL 60661
(312) 440-2500

American Diabetes Association
1660 Duke Street
Alexandria, VA 22314
(703) 549-1500

American Foundation for the
Blind
15 West 16th Street
New York, NY 10011
(800) 232-5463

American Heart Association
7272 Greenville Avenue
Dallas, TX 75231
(214) 373-6300

American Hospital Association
840 North Lake Shore Drive
Chicago, IL 60611
(312) 280-6000

American Lung Association
1740 North Broadway
New York, NY 10019
(212) 315-8700

American Medical Association
535 North State Street
Chicago, IL 60610
(312) 464-5000

American Public Health
Association
1015 15th Street NW
Washington, DC 20006
(202) 789-5600

American Red Cross
1730 D Street NW
Washington, DC 20006
(202) 434-4074

Centers for Disease Control and
Prevention
1600 Clifton Road NE
Atlanta, GA 30333
(404) 639-3311

Family Health Foundation Library
1740 West 92nd Street
Kansas City, MO 64114
(816) 333-9700

HEALTH PROMOTION
Association for Worksite Health
Promotion
60 Revere Drive
Suite 500
Northbrook, Illinois 60062
(708) 480-9574

National Wellness Association
University of Wisconsin, Stevens
Point
Stevens Point, WI 54481
(715) 346-2172

Office of Disease Prevention and
Health Promotion
Room 2132, Switzer Building
330 C Street SW
Washington, DC 20201
(202) 472-5660

The Wellness Councils of America
1823 Garbet Street, Suite 201
Omaha, Nebraska 68102
(402) 444-1711

INFANT HEALTH
Division of Maternal, Infant and
Adolescent Health
Parklawn Building, Room 18A-30
5600 Fishers Lane
Rockville, MD 20857
(301) 443-2250

INSURANCE
Consumers Union
2001 S Street NW, Suite 520
Washington, DC 20009
(202) 462-6262

Health Insurance Association of
America
1025 Connecticut Avenue NW
Washington, DC 20036
(800) 635-1271

MENTAL HEALTH/STRESS
American Institute of Stress
124 Park Avenue
Yonkers, NY 10703
(914) 963-1200

Employee Assistance Professional
Association
4601 N. Fairfax Drive, Suite 1001
Arlington, VA 22203
(703) 522-6272

National Mental Health
Association
1021 Prince Street
Alexandria, VA 22314
(800) 969-6642

NUTRITION
Food and Nutrition Information
Center
Department of Agriculture
National Agricultural Library,
Room 304
Beltsville, MD 20705
(301) 504-5719

National Dairy Council
10255 W. Higgins, Suite 900
Rosemont, IL 60018
(708) 803-2000

ON-LINE COMPUTER SERVICES
*America Online: Better Health &
Medical Forum.* For free software
and trial time call: 1-800-827-
6364, ext. 6751.

Prodigy. Contact your local software or computer retailer.
(914) 993-8843.

INFORMED Resources

SAFETY

National Safety Council
444 North Michigan Avenue
Chicago, IL 60611
(708) 285-1121

National Institute of Occupational
Safety and Health (NIOSH)
4676 Columbia Parkway
Cincinnati, OH 45226
(800) 35-NIOSH

National Highway Traffic Safety
Administration
400 7th Street SW, Room 5118
Washington, DC 20590
(800) 424-9393

SELF-CARE BOOKS

*Before You Call The Doctor: Safe ,
Effective Self-Care for Over 300
Common Medical Problems,* by
Anne Simons, M.D. et al, New
York: Fawcett Columbine, 1992.

Healthwise Handbook, by Donald
W. Kemper. Boise, Idaho:
Healthwise, Inc., 1991.

*House Calls: How Doctors Treat
Themselves and Their Own Families
for Common Illnesses and Injuries,*
by Gerald Cousens, New York:
Fireside, 1993.

*Take Care of Yourself: Your
Personal Guide to Self-Care and
Preventing Illness,* by Donald M.
Vickery, M.D., and James Fries,
M.D. Reading, Mass.: Addison-
Wesley, 1993.

*The American Medical Association
Family Health Guide,* Jeffrey R.M.
Kunz, M.D., and Asher J. Finkel,
M.D. eds., New York: Random
House, 1987.

*The PDR Family Guide To
Prescription Drugs,* Monvale, New
Jersey: Medical Economics Data,
1993.

*WorkCare: A Resource Guide for the
Working Person,* by George J.
Pfeiffer and Judith A. Webster,
Charlottesville, Virginia:
WorkCare Press, 1992.

SELF-CARE NEWSLETTERS:

Harvard Health Letter, published
by Harvard Medical School
Health Publications Group, 164
Longwood Avenue, Boston, MA
02115

Nutrition Action Health Letter, published by Center for Science in
the Public Interest, Suite 300,
1875 Connecticut Ave.,
Washington, D.C. 20009-5728

Tufts University & Nutrition Letter,
published by Tufts University,
203 Harrison Ave., Boston, MA

*University of California at Berkeley
Wellness Letter,* published by
Health Letter Associates, P.O. Box
420148, Palm Coast, FL, 32142

Work & Life Newsletter, published
by the WorkCare Group, P.O.
Box 2053, Charlottesville, VA,
22902 (804) 977-7525

INDEX

INDEX

J

Joint flexibility, 82
    injury, 80-88
    tendonitis, 84-85, 87-88

K

Kidney disease, 98
Knee pain, 87

L

Life departments, 16
Lyme disease, 77, 80
Lymph glands, 58-59, 117

M

Mammography, 20
Marijuana, 108
Maximum dollar limit, 25
Medical self-care, 4
Medical tests, 19
Medications, see Drugs
Medicine chest
    home, 47
Melanoma, 73
Menstrual cramps, 89
Migraine headaches, 94
Money, saving, 39
Mumps, 59
Muscle strains, 82

N

Narcotics, 107
Neck pain, 83
Nutrition
    "Five-A-Day Plan," 6, 10
    Food Pyramid, 11

O

Obesity, 6, 13, 100, 101, 111
Occult blood, testing, 19
Office visit, 28
Out-of-pocket maximum for
    health insurance, 25
Opiates, 107
Options—treatment, 30, 34, 37
Over-the-counter medications, 50

P

Pap smear, 20

Patient's rights, 41
Periodontal disease, 64
Physical activity, 6, 8-9
Physician
    choosing, 26-27
    INFORMED Process, 34-37
    INFORMED Worksheet, 35
    Primary Care Physician, 26-27
    questions to ask, 26, 30, 34-37
    talking to, 30
Poisoning, 46
Poison Ivy, 76
Pre-certification review, 25
Preferred provider
    organization (PPO), 25
Pregnancy, planning, 111
Premenstrual Syndrome, 90
Preterm labor, preventing, 113
Prevention, "Building Blocks," 6
Proteins, 10
Prostate, 20, 92
Puncture wounds, 72
Pyramid, food, 11

R

Reasonable and customary, 25
Relaxation
    techniques, 17
    walking, 18
Reye's syndrome, preventing, 51
Risks—treatment, 30, 34-37

S

Second opinion, 30
Sedatives, 107
Sexually transmitted disease, 91,
    92, 111, 117
Shortness of breath, 65-66
Sigmoidoscopy, 20
Skin abrasions, 70
Skin cancer, 7, 73
Sleep, 95
Smoking, 6-7, 53, 61
Sodium, 10, 98
Sore throat, 54
Stimulants, 107
Stomach flu, 67
Stress
    identifying, 15

    management skills, 15-16
    relaxation, 17-18
Sugar, 10-12
Surgery, questions to ask, 34, 38
Swollen glands, 59

T

Tendonitis, 84
Tension headaches, 93
Tetanus shots, 21, 70-72
Travel
    medical emergency, 45
Treatment
    home care, 51-52
    options, 34-37
    questions to ask your
    doctor, 30, 34-37

U

Ulcers, 65
Urinary problems, 92

V

Vaginitis, 91

W

Walking, 8
Warm-up, 82
Water, 51
Weight management, 13
Wrist pain, 85

X

X-rays
    dental, 19, 64

Y

Yeast infections, 91

128